# THE FOUNTAIN

# THE
# FOUNTAIN

## A DOCTOR'S PRESCRIPTION TO MAKE
## 60
## THE NEW
## 30

## DR. ROCCO MONTO
FOREWORD BY BILL MAHER

RODALE.

# RODALE *wellness*

*Live happy. Be healthy. Get inspired.*

Sign up today to get exclusive access to our authors, exclusive bonuses, and the most authoritative, useful, and cutting-edge information on health, wellness, fitness, and living your life to the fullest.

**Visit us online at RodaleWellness.com**
**Join us at RodaleWellness.com/Join**

Printed in the United States of America

Rodale Inc. makes every effort to use acid-free ∞, recycled paper ♻.

Illustrations by Jacob Scheyder

Book design by Jordan Wannemacher

Library of Congress Cataloging-in-Publication Data is on file with the publisher.

ISBN 978–1–63565–233–8

Distributed to the trade by Macmillan

2  4  6  8  10  9  7  5  3  1  hardcover

# ☘ RODALE.

We inspire health, healing, happiness, and love in the world.
Starting with you.

*To my wife, Jennifer, for making me want to live forever.*

*To my kids, Rocky, Siena, Nick, and Alex, for supporting me when I do.*

# CONTENTS

*Foreword by Bill Maher*      ix

*Introduction: Proof of Concept*      xi


## PHASE ONE: SCIENCE

1. The Hunt for the Aging Off-Button      3
2. The Crucible      19
3. Ancient Invaders      39
4. The 4-Hour Rule      49
5. Hacking the Genome      57


## PHASE TWO: DIET

6. Bridge of Lies      69
7. A High-Steaks Game      92
8. Green Is the New Black      101
9. Supplement City      111

## PHASE THREE: EXERCISE AND MIND-BODY

10. Harder, Better, Faster, Younger                     131
11. The Catalyst                                        140
12. The Tao of Aging                                    149
13. Agents of Change                                    158

## PHASE FOUR: MEDS

14. Better Living through Chemistry                     169
15. Blinded by Science                                  183
16. Stranger Things                                     189

## PHASE FIVE: THE PLAN

17. The Fountain Plan                                   203

Acknowledgments                                         213
Glossary                                                215
Endnotes                                                219
Index                                                   259

# FOREWORD
## BY BILL MAHER

I'M WRITING THIS FOREWORD because I really think Dr. Monto is on to something in the way he breaks down the intricacies of the confusing medical world we're confronted with, toward the purpose of living longer and healthier lives. And as I'm now 61, this is of great interest to me!

I am a believer that humans are in the infancy of their understanding of the human body and how it works, but Rocco at least seems to be trying. That's another reason I liked this book: I found something so rare . . . a doctor with humility. Also, the book seems very science based, not just medical-science based. As I was reading this book, I just kept thinking, *Boy, this guy really lives to figure this stuff out.* Which would be great! Did I mention I was 61?

I also think this book will make some other doctors angry, and that's good. It's so easy for ideas, even bad ideas, to calcify into conventional wisdom. Look at poor fat. It never really was the bad guy, but for a while it was really on the outs! Just the worst stuff in the world. Then what? It changed? No, we just saw things differently. We came to our senses. Come home, fat, all is forgiven. I'm just a layman, but stuff like that makes me think, *Can't we do things more scientifically?*

There's so much faddism in the medical talk that reaches us in books and through doctors talking on TV. I remember in the early 1970s there was controversy and a lot of talk about the influx of "preservatives"—ooh, there are too many preservatives in the food! It was a big subject for 10 minutes, and then everyone went, "This Sara Lee shortcake is delicious!" But I swear I remember America pausing for a hot minute and asking, "Should we really be making this big a departure from the food we think of as *off the farm*?"

For me to trust a doctor, he or she can't be the kind who never even asks you what you eat. And he or she has to always be interested in what is causing the symptoms, not just in making the symptoms go away. For example, I used to use nasal spray, and now I think back in horror—a product specifically designed to only treat the symptom by pushing the toxic gunk coming out of me *back into my body*! It's such a perfect metaphor for so much of the American way of dealing with disease.

But not in these pages. This doctor-author? He's a surgeon who doesn't want to have to do surgery—kind of the way it's always the generals who've been to war who don't want to fight another one. I don't want to "do" surgery either.

I am far from a perfect practitioner of all the smart advice in this book, but it's a victory of sorts just to know when and how much I'm really cheating. No one respects more than I do the individual's right to decide for himself or herself how much of their own health they want to trade for pleasure. I always just wanted to know where the goalposts were!

I always said about health, whenever the subject came up at a cocktail party, "You gotta win the battle on the molecular level." So true, so true. And this book really helped me understand what the hell I ever meant by that.

# INTRODUCTION
## PROOF OF CONCEPT

"We go through life. We shed our skins. We become ourselves.
Ultimately, we are not seeking others to bow to, but to reinforce our
individual natures, to help us suffer our own choices, to guide us
on our own particular journeys."

—PATTI SMITH, *DETAILS*, 1993

**I AM AFRAID OF** dying. It's not the beginning or middle of life that is the
problem; it's the end. Those last 10 years have me scared. You see, getting
older is a relatively new thing, and the fact is that we really aren't that good
at it. To be sure, medicine has done a great job over the past century helping
us all live longer. Clean water, antibiotics, and modern surgery have post-
poned checkout time for most of us. The problem is that while life span has
increased, our *health span* hasn't kept pace. I am an orthopedic surgeon,
and I will be the first to admit to you that contemporary healthcare has
created a generation of invalids—people just surviving, not thriving, at the
end of their lives. Our parents, who worked their whole lives for a retirement they thought would be filled with joy and purpose, are withering away
as their frail bodies and minds disintegrate. Heart disease, hypertension,

strokes, renal disease, diabetes, and fractures are more common than ever. Rates of Alzheimer's disease, Parkinson's, and depression are rising. Doctors continue to treat the symptoms while the causes go unmanaged. Aging has become unsustainable.

The sad part of all this is that we didn't just screw over one generation. We took down two. I see this all the time in my office, devoted daughters and sons sacrificing their emotional and financial resources to try to deal with the unintentional but escalating demands of their parents' failing health and vitality. Worse than that, they see what is happening to their parents and wonder what fate has in store for them. Add a dash of obesity and a touch of desperation, and you have a heady mix that makes people feel powerless and fatigued. Rudderless in a white water they can't control. Two generations twisting in a medical, economic, and social whirlpool that is draining the vitality of our families and nation. Well I say, to hell with that.

I am a baby boomer. You know, the generation that blew up every demographic we passed through like a pig in a python. Well, we're coming around the final clubhouse turn and heading for the Big Finale. Every day 10,000 people turn 60. Every single day. By 2050, the global population over 60 will double to more than two billion people. This trend has been called a silver tsunami, and the staggering medical needs that accompany this wave are expected to push our yearly national healthcare bill here in the United States to more than $4 trillion by 2030.

If we fail to make the changes needed to address the coming wave, it will not be for lack of funds. The global market for anti-aging products is increasing by 8 percent per year and will reach $191.7 billion by 2019. Insurance companies and Big Pharma have focused on drug pipelines responding to symptoms instead of causes and have been rewarded with handsome profits. The new millennium has seen a radical shift in our cultural attitude toward aging, and longevity research has exploded during the last 3 years. Still not convinced? Google certainly is. Its new life extension venture, Calico (a division of Alphabet), has put their money where their big data is. They inked a $1.5 billion 10-year joint deal with the Chicago-based pharmaceutical giant AbbVie to develop a new line of anti-aging drugs and therapies. Hungry startups abound in this new anti-aging galaxy. Unity

Biotechnology, a maker of senolytic medications to reverse heart disease, osteoarthritis, and failing eyesight, has raised $116 million in Series B funding. The investors include Jeff Bezos and the investment arm of Amazon, Bezos Expeditions. Even the FDA, who had never previously acknowledged aging as a disease process, has finally shifted gears. This year the FDA approved its first-ever anti-aging drug study, a clinical trial of metformin.

It's not just the AARP-crowd that is grappling with growing old. Who are the biggest consumers of plastic surgery in the United States? The Gen Xers. The generation known for extending adolescence is now hoping to extend their lives, too. They don't just want to age healthier, they want to age prettier. Gen Xers are consuming anti-aging products and supplements at a record clip. Next up, the Millennials—a generation that craves authoritative, doctor-endorsed products is now seeking innovative solutions for healthy, experiential living. People of every age are looking for the pathways to better aging.

But what if the solutions were already here? What if we could translate all the exotic science and research breakthroughs of today into a practical plan that could invigorate and energize the way we all live right now? What if there were already ways to ease the negative effects of aging and keep diabetes, heart disease, cancer, Parkinson's disease, and Alzheimer's disease from ever starting? What if we could win the war on aging through prevention instead of intervention? I don't know about you, but I am determined not to repeat the mistakes of the past and be herded to the north forty to run out the clock. I don't just want to go through the motions. I want to thrive. And I think you do, too. You just need the tools. Where will you find the knowledge, instruction, advice, and motivation to get this difficult job done? Right here. Right now.

*The Fountain* is the story of a relationship—the most intense and complex relationship of all: the one between your body and your environment. Like all affairs, it's defined by choices and sacrifice. Decisions carry consequences. Freedom demands responsibility. For most people, this relationship has always been unbalanced. Asymmetric. No matter what you do, it seems impossible to level the field. Our leaders have kept us in the dark, and those we have trusted most, our caregivers, are only now beginning to shed their white coats and partner with us. Not anymore. *The Fountain* is meant to be disruptive. It questions the established doctrines of traditional medicine that have brought us to this tipping point. This book is intended to give you the knowledge and tools to begin to recalibrate your approach to health. It will empower you to take control of your life and make better choices. It was written to help you thrive.

The book is organized into five distinct sections. I call them phases. Each section stands on its own, so cruise around as you like. You can pit for gas anytime. Anywhere. Phase One covers the science of aging. Science is, by definition, the art of observation. The opening chapter starts with the observation that the world is sprinkled with anti-aging hot spots, places where people have been able to live longer and more vigorous lives than anywhere else. Why start there? Because science requires context. Before you start drilling down to the microcellular level, you need to gain some perspective. People who live in these areas, called blue zones, which include Sardinia, Okinawa, Ikaria, Nicoya, and Loma Linda, have average life spans that exceed the rest of the world by at least 10 years. Not too shabby. More importantly, people who live in the blue zones have less chronic disease and more active lives. What do these widely disparate locales, some of them achingly isolated and rugged, possibly have in common that binds them together in a battle for vitality and longevity? There are clues. People in the blue zones eat a plant-based diet, rarely retire, exercise vigorously, and live with faith and purpose. What does this tell us? Humans are a resilient, ingenious species, and challenging environments select for the toughest of us. Check. You could take the blue pill and you'd probably be fine, but you would never know why. You'll just go on believing what you choose to believe. Don't do it. Take the red pill and keep reading, it will be worth it.

The first phase of the book also focuses on the fascinating science of aging. In this section, you will learn about what the brilliant Spanish biologist Carlos López-Otín and his colleagues call the hallmarks of aging. This team has created the first true unified model of metabolism, and it is all about energy and error. We'll review each of these seven hallmarks, or signs, and their unique characteristics, and you'll learn how to harness this incredible research to improve the quality of your health and life.

Can you cheat death? Not yet. But you can scam the hell out of life. *The Fountain* surveys the latest research on diet, exercise, mindfulness, supplements, and medications specifically targeted to help you wring the most out of life and to make the whole thing worth it.

The science section, and really, the rest of the book, is all about giving you the practical information and tactics you need to win these metabolic duels. Decrease error and preserve energy. You'll learn how mitochondria work and why they are so critical to our vitality. If you're going to live longer, you are going to need some more gas in the tank to get the job done. Nicotinamide adenosine dinucleotide (NAD+) molecules are your factory's fuel rods and the most precious biochemical commodities in the metabolic universe. NAD+ is both the hammer and chisel of life. It is an important cofactor in many enzymatic processes and a critical player in generating the fuel to run those reactions. If you take one lesson home from this book, remember the importance of NAD+. I'll also introduce some ways to keep your NAD+ levels high through exercise, diet, and supplements. Think stem cells and gene editing will hook you up with some sparkling new virgin DNA? Sorry, but you can't get a genetic face-lift just yet. For now, you will have to be content with doing it the hard way. I will show you the risks and benefits of fasting and caloric restriction and why people can't stick to it (hint: you already know why). Fasting works, but it is brutal on active people, and it simply isn't a very practical approach to longevity. There are more attractive alternatives. You'll also discover your first dietary tool to live healthier—time-restricted feeding (TRF). By limiting all your meals to within 12 hours or fewer, you can leverage the influence of your natural circadian rhythms and delay many of the hallmarks of aging.

The next phase in the book is diet, and things get serious here. *The Fountain* questions authority and undermines medical dogma with facts. We'll bust all the biggest dietary myths. We've been told for 40 years that saturated fat causes high cholesterol, and high cholesterol causes heart disease. Nonsense. The diet-heart hypothesis is not supported by most research. Heart disease is driven by inflammation. You can get up to 35 percent of your daily calories from fat and mix the saturation level any way your little sclerotic-free heart wants to. Well, then sugar is going to kill you, right? Wrong, sort of. Overeating is going to kill you, not glucose. Your mitochondria need glucose to make ATP, the energy currency of the body. Sugar will just make your slow-motion suicide a little less painful. Look, you can get up to 55 percent of your calories from carbohydrates and you'll do just fine. Keep the sugar at 5 percent. This won't be that crazy hard if you avoid the place where most sugar is burrowed—deep within processed food. It's lying in wait in your bag of Doritos for a chance to punch a ticket straight to your bliss point. Salt is another misunderstood thing. Where is most of Na+? Right next to the sugar in your party bag of chips. Once you get rid of the processed foods, the amount of dietary salt in your diet crashes down. If you continually load up your diet with salt, high levels might eventually hurt you by causing osteoporosis or cancer. What else can salt do? Adding salt to your food makes you hungry, not thirsty.

Don't get me started on gluten-free. If you have celiac disease, I am so sorry because that sucks for you incredibly. It is a terrible autoimmune condition that reaches far beyond issues of gluten and wheat. As for gluten sensitivity, I am not buying it just yet. You'll have to prove that one to me. Hey, I say go gluten-free if you think it makes you feel better, but beware of the very real risks of mercury and arsenic poisoning from a gluten-free diet. Rice is the original toxin sponge. Don't believe me? Skip on over to Chapter 6 and find out the hidden dangers of going G-free. You can also amaze your friends and read about what gluten is. When you're done, you can go grab some guilt-free pizza.

You could say that you don't eat pizza because you're on a high-protein diet. If you are, you need to shoot over to Chapter 7 to read up on why that might not be the brightest move ever. Protein itself is not bad, but an average guy needs only around 56 grams a day to take care of normal cellular maintenance, including muscle repair. The average gal needs even less; about 46 grams a day will keep her system humming. High protein intake is fine when you're growing or if you're a young athlete in the middle of a heavy training regimen. However, long-term high-protein diets do two very bad things. One, they can overload the filtration system in your kidneys. Two, they push up your levels of insulin-like growth factor-1 (IGF-1). Think that's great? You shouldn't, because IGF-1 is like catnip for cancer.

Don't worry, I didn't skip over any protected dietary classifications in my research for this book. In Chapter 8 I try to wrap my delicate stems around what being a vegan really means. Vegans reap some real benefits beyond identity and politics. Strength and physical performance are not incompatible with a life without meat. There are many great athletes who live off the green stuff alone. Remember that all choices carry consequences. The bottom line is that plant-based diets are cool, but we were designed as omnivores. If you are going to pull off the whole vegan lifestyle and stick with it, you better have your Amazon Dash button preloaded for regular vitamin $B_{12}$ and iron supplements. Can you say vegetanemia?

The diet phase of *The Fountain* does wrap up with some good news: Coffee and tea are back, baby. Supplements are the aperitifs in this section, and I will help you to make some sense out of the absolute hot mess of literature on this controversial topic. The most important lesson of this chapter is that you should accept the fact that most of the world today is vitamin D deficient. Optimizing your vitamin D levels will help you maintain your bones and connective tissues. It also does a good job of mopping up excess circulating IGF-1 to lower the risk of cancer. In fact, when you get done whipping through this introduction, the first thing you should do is to roll on over to a pharmacy and buy yourself a bottle of vitamin $D_3$ supplements. Your future self will thank you for it.

The next step in your journey is Phase Three: Exercise and Mind-Body. Of all the tools to combat the crappy way we age, exercise is the most powerful. There is no food, pill, or procedure that affects the body as powerfully as exercise. It truly is medicine. Working out alters the histone arrangements and epigenetic profile of your DNA within minutes. It improves your insulin sensitivity and energy reserves. It decelerates every hallmark of aging and promotes vitality. It is also sweaty and difficult. You need about 1 hour a day to get the job done. The type of exercise you choose is far less important than the simple act of doing it. I have my favorites, and you'll learn why there really is no gain without a little pain. BTW, sweating is not an indication of caloric burn. It is simply a means to dissipate excess body heat. Hey, we can do some vinyasas together as you learn more about the benefits of yoga, tai chi, and other types of qigong. Wax on, wax off, people.

The final aspect of the exercise phase of *The Fountain* is all about getting your mental groove on. Let's face it, getting older is not for the faint of heart. Mental focus and clarity will buy you some more time and help you stay sharp. Are Web-based mental training sites worth the money? No. I do believe in the concept of flow and think that people get more creative as they get older. The biggest mental advantage you could ever have to gain longevity is a strong sense of purpose. Never retire. Ever. Don't move into an assisted living facility or retirement home. Ever. Your mind needs stimulation, and there is a natural affinity between the young and old that is too frequently ignored. If you want to live longer and keep the nugget working, you need to demand attention and interaction. Still, modern life is noisy. It's important to get comfortable with silence and reconnect with your thoughts. Ten minutes of meditation a day is all you need to enhance creativity and performance no matter what your age.

I know what you're thinking. This whole Fountain thing sounds awfully involved. Diet, exercise, supplements, meditation. Isn't there some kind of pill that I can take that can do all this stuff for me, doc? Well . . . I wondered the same thing. We might not be there yet, but we aren't that far from offering useful anti-aging drugs. I devote Phase Four to the medications that are being evaluated to help us live longer and better. As you reach midlife, your body starts to slow down its production of most of the hormones that define your personality and sexuality. The big four players here are testosterone, estrogen, growth hormone, and oxytocin. The real deal is that if you're a middle-aged man and feeling crappy, it doesn't hurt to get your free testosterone level checked. You're probably okay, but when you are having trouble in the sack, the mind has a way of magnifying the problem. If you do have low T, there is nothing wrong with trialling low-dose supplements to nudge you back to the normal range. It doesn't appear to elevate your risk of prostate cancer, although I would avoid supplementing if I had a history of prostate cancer. It might not turn your bedroom into a game of Twister, but it couldn't hurt. If you do take a trip on the T train, please do it with a real live doctor watching your blood levels, not on your own through some sketchy dark web Italian pharmacy. Lei capisce? Hint: If you find that you have anger management issues, you might want to lay off the androgens and just stick to eggs and bacon.

Ladies, an increasing body of research suggests you should consider a few years of transdermal estrogen replacement therapy after you reach menopause if you've had a hysterectomy. No hysterectomy? Then let symptoms be your guide. Clearly, you can't go the estrogen route if you've had breast cancer, particularly if it was an estrogen-positive tumor. Some of the difficult symptoms of menopause that women face are hot flashes and night sweats, which can wreck your sleep. Estrogen replacement can help, or you could also consider bioidenticals of selective serotonin reuptake inhibitors. Anyway, you'll want to read this section before you talk to your doctor. It will help you get a handle on the realistic risks and benefits of this approach.

As for growth hormone supplementation, there is no doubt it does have a positive impact on lean body mass and muscle size in both men and women. But there is a huge downside. I recommend steering clear of growth hormone therapy as you get older because of the very real risk that its elevation of circulating IGF-1 will promote cancer development. It can also cause diabetes and heart problems. Oxytocin is a psychoactive hormone that seems to affect vitality. There is a lot of interest now in this hormone, and it may prove to be helpful in preventing frailty in the elderly. I'm listening.

Why do you need this book? Because it works. And perhaps you've reached the point where you've realized you need to make a change. I am a perfect example of how life can wear you down and lead you to a tipping point. Mine came at the hands of a surly, meaty-handed male nurse. Wait. I probably should explain. A few years ago, I thought I was doing pretty well. A busy practice on the beautiful island of Nantucket, two freshly minted children, and a beautiful wife. But there were some cracks in my foundation. I was having trouble keeping up my practice, my energy was low, my joints ached, and my wife was getting tired of my constant complaining. I felt terrible, but I blamed everybody else for my state. I never thought the problem could actually be me.

When I started having some weird neck and arm pain, I became alarmed. In true doctor fashion, I called my insurance agent to check on my disability coverage rather than seeing a physician. My agent lives in Philadelphia, and I hadn't seen him in 20 years. He thought I needed more disability insurance (of course) and that I just needed an exam. He arranged for somebody to come out to the island to check me out. A few days later, a nurse from the insurance company made landfall and came by the office to do a physical exam. I unbuttoned my shirt and laid down on my crinkling table paper while this big, sweaty male nurse did an EKG on me. He casually asked me how tall I was. "Five-foot-10," I told him. He raised an eyebrow. Then he asked how much I weighed. I said what I always say when the nice ladies check me in for my inter-island Cessna flights—185. He laughed and told me that may have been what I used to weigh. I persisted. "No, I'm 185, I'm what I've always been." He tipped his smudged glasses down his nose and challenged me to use my scale or his. I chose the home-field advantage scale. 210. Two hundred and ten pounds. Shocked, I think I must have jiggled a little as I slowly sat down. I guess my wife wasn't shrinking my pants in the dryer. The nurse, who was easily twice my jumbo size, drew some blood from my fluffy veins and packed up his gear. "You'll be hearing from us," he said as he left. Great.

My insurance guy called me a couple of days later. He wanted to know what the hell had happened to me. He asked me when I got old and fat. Nice. Then he tried to make me feel better and told me that he might be able to get me some insurance but that it was going to cost me. I had already stopped listening. *What happened to you, Rock? When did you get old and fat?*

Look, I've been an athlete all my life, and I'm a surgeon. Vain, self-centered, and more than a little egotistical. No argument there. Old and fat, however, was not acceptable. So, I started doing everything I had always been taught in medicine about living healthfully. I went on a low-fat, high-protein diet, started playing soccer once a week again, and cut out the snacks. I even ate apples. Apples! Six weeks later, still feeling cruddy, but a little leaner, I got on the scale for my triumphant exoneration. The scale spun like a roulette wheel. 208. I rubbed my eyes and jiggled a little while I double-checked the number. 208. My wife, who is ridiculously fit and insists on working out every day, told me I was doing it all wrong. I had to exercise every day, I had to eat less, and I needed to be less obsessive. Yeah, I got that. Sometimes I can be a little slow on the uptake, but I did realize that I needed to find a different way. I just wanted to know why. I started reading and researching everything I could get my hands on. The more I learned, the more I realized that she was right. I asked my wife for one of her workout DVDs. She gave me an "easy one." I thought I was going to die, but I did it. I started doing daily high-intensity interval training. The workouts slowly got easier. I went to a balanced diet, cut down the calories, and started eating all my meals within a 10-hour period.

Things started happening fast. Good things. The weight started coming off. After 2 weeks, I lost 8 pounds. By 1 month, I had lost 15 and gave my wife permission to start throwing my pants in the dryer again. After 2 months, I had lost 25 pounds. At 3 months, my weight crept back up a little, but I realized that I could fool my internal thermostat by varying my diet and the type and length of my exercise. At 6 months, I was down to 180 pounds and felt a helluva lot better about everything.

That was 5 years ago, and I'm still 30 pounds lighter and feel 30 years younger than I did then. I've incorporated all the lessons I learned into *The Fountain,* and with this book in your hands, you, too, have the tools to look and feel much younger than you ever thought you could. You don't have to be an athlete or medical person to do what I did. You just need some knowledge, motivation, and a little discipline to pull it off. It's not crazy hard. It's a tactical approach backed by intense scientific research. Eating better, eating less. Working out more, working out smarter. Taking targeted supplements. Using medications to fix the rest. Restoring the balance between mind, body, and environment. Does it require some work? Damned right it does, but the results will be worth it.

What if you're only 30 or 40? I have news for you. Your DNA doesn't care. You need to start applying the lessons in this book ASAP if you want to change your molecular fate. If you are serious about staying healthy, it doesn't matter whether you are 20, 30, 40, 50, or 60. Your environment and lifestyle are already scrambling your genetic profile. If you are over 60, the clock is ticking. You better pay close attention and start your genetic renovation project immediately. Given enough time, most damage can be reversed. And time is the essence of this book.

That's how *The Fountain* flows. Think of it as an owner's guide to your body. A Google Maps to help you make better choices about how you live every day. When you are finished reading this book, it will all begin to make sense. There is no one single answer to the aging question. The solutions are complex. Yet, there is an elegance in their connectivity; a beauty in the science of it all. Metabolism is the network that connects diet, exercise, supplements, and medication. The sooner you learn the floor plan, the better. *The Fountain* won't provide every answer you're seeking, but it will give you a scaffold to frame the right questions. I might still be afraid of dying, but after researching and writing this book, I gained a clarity and vision about aging that I never had before. I used to fear getting older, but I am not afraid anymore. After you read this book, you won't be either. We are going to crush this thing together.

What is an orthopedic surgeon like me doing talking about aging? One reason is that my work takes me right through ground zero of the very worst things that aging can do to people. Terrible things. I've spent my entire career rebuilding the worn-out cartilage, ripped tendons, and shattered bones that result from the way we have always aged. A surgical sin-eater. A collector. But it doesn't have to be like this. Any one of the tools in this book can help turn this rusty freighter around and make aging a graceful and rewarding trek. Put them all together, and senior life starts looking a whole lot more junior. Don't let the slippage of time simply mold you. Make health a habit. If you start applying the lessons you learn in *The Fountain* now, you won't just have a better tomorrow, you'll have a better today.

The other reason I am here telling you about aging is that I am a translator. I spend most of my day turning complex, scary situations into understandable, scalable explanations. The world can be a dark, dangerous place. Lighting it properly takes patience, nuance, and a keen interest in not just the why, but the how.

*The Fountain* is the product of years of canvassing the world for the latest meaningful opinions on longevity and thousands of hours spent reviewing and curating primary scientific research, and it will take you from the exotic corners of the globe to the churning nucleus of our cells, from sterile laboratories to sweaty gyms, from heights of outer space to depths of inner space. What are you waiting for? The secrets of a long life full of health, vitality, and meaning await.

# PHASE ONE
## SCIENCE

# 1

# THE HUNT FOR THE AGING OFF-BUTTON

"The longer I live, the more beautiful life becomes."
—FRANK LLOYD WRIGHT, 1958

**THE DESIRE TO LIVE** longer and healthier has always been a part of what makes us human. Tales of exotic lands where people live long, blissful lives without sickness have drawn explorers for thousands of years. Shambhala. P'eng-lai. Bimini. The Fountain of Youth. Every culture has a mythological land that it identifies with immortality. Modern myths of longevity have now drawn a whole new breed of explorers. Epidemiologists, geneticists, pharmacologists, and biologists have replaced the adventurers of the past. Today they are seeking answers to the secrets of aging that are hiding in plain sight. For decades, researchers have known that there are regions scattered around the world where people live much longer than expected. Starting in the remote mountains of central Sardinia, Belgian demographer Michel Poulain and Italian physician-researcher Gianni Pes spent years carefully identifying and cataloging these extraordinary groups of centenarians.[1] After every new discovery of a longevity hot spot, they would circle the area on a world map in blue marker. These "blue zones" were later popularized by their collaborator, journalist Dan Buettner, in a series of books and documentaries supported in part by the National Geographic Society.[2, 3]

These longevity zones now include Okinawa (Japan), Sardinia (Italy), Ikaria (Greece), Nicoya (Costa Rica), and Loma Linda (United States). People living in these communities have an average life span of 89 years compared to 79 years for the rest of the world. What possible connections could link Italian sheepherders, Japanese grandmothers, Greek grandfathers, Costa Rican farmers, and suburban Californian Seventh-Day Adventists? Are they diaspora from a long-forgotten homeland of immortals that share some secret genetic code? Is their extreme longevity simply a function of healthy diet and lifestyle? Or is it, as my father-in-law says, just damn good luck?

Tantalizing clues to these mysteries are emerging as scientists scour the health histories, migration patterns, diet, and genetics of the world's blue zones. All this demographic data has resulted in more questions than answers, but some common themes are taking shape. Many of the elderly residents of these areas share a calorie-restricted and plant-based diet, a slow pace of life, intense physical exercise, purposeful work, and a supportive network of family and friends. It is only now that we are beginning to understand how this unique blend of diet, fitness, and emotional support leads to direct changes in the genome that might slow down our internal aging clocks. Special places make special people.

## OUT OF TIME AND HISTORY[4]

The story of the blue zones starts on the rocky island of Sardinia, 222 miles off the west coast of Italy across the aquamarine Tyrrhenian Sea. The second-largest isle in the Mediterranean Sea (9,300 square miles) and one of the oldest land masses in Europe, Sardinia has been continuously inhabited since the Paleolithic period. Repeatedly invaded, occupied, and colonized throughout its history, Sardinia is ever defiant. It remains culturally, socially, and genetically distinct from the rest of Italy. Even its native language, Sard, is unique and considered the closest to Latin in the world. The emerald ring of water that surrounds Sardinia encloses two very different worlds. Most of the island's 1.6 million residents live near its sandy coastlines, hosting more than 10 million tourists per year. However, it is the secluded population of the central mountain ranges that has drawn intense interest from scientists studying longevity.

Isolated by imposing terrain like Punta la Marmora, the island's highest peak at more than 6,000 feet, the people of the remote upland Nuoro province live "like birds in the sky."[5] They still herd the island's four million sheep (more than New Zealand) and typically walk more than 5 miles a day along the massifs and ravines to get supplies for their families. These central Sardinians have always been known for their melancholy, rugged character and long life spans.

Sardinia's history is entwined with Greek mythology. An island where men and gods once shared the same volcanic lands. An island where truth and legend have always mixed freely. It was modern stories of centenarian hot spots that first drew the attention of Gianni Pes more than 20 years ago. Pes was meticulously detailed in his survey. He visited every one of 377 municipalities to confirm the local stories of longevity pockets. The estimated life expectancy in the mountainous center of the island was indeed much higher than in other areas of the world. There are 21 people more than 100 years old for every 10,000 in these villages, compared to only 1.73 per 10,000 in the United States.[6] Men live longer than anywhere else on Earth. The male to female ratio among locally born centenarians is 1.35 compared to 2.43 in the rest of Sardinia. Sorry fellas, but here in the States women have a five times greater chance of hitting the century mark than we do. The demographic research also yielded some good news for me. Shorter Sard men tend to live 2 years longer than taller men. Sweet news for us diminutive Neapolitans.

Sardinians often greet each other with the traditional phrase *a kent'an-nos,* meaning "may you live to a hundred." Their traditional diet is high in complex carbohydrates punctuated by grass-fed goat and sheep milk and cheese. The Sardinians eat 15 pounds of this cheese rich in omega-3 fatty acids every year. If you think that sounds heavy, Americans knock down 35 pounds of mostly corn-fed derived cheese a year. A unique island delicacy is the larvae-laced sheep's milk cheese casu marzu, usually smeared with eucalyptus honey and rumored to be an aphrodisiac. Some more Sardinian fly, my love?

Although they don't eat a calorie-restricted diet, the oldest Sards have lived through decades of famine due to war, poverty, and disease. Their meat intake is generally limited to once or twice a week. Flatbread, fava beans, fish, fennel, tomatoes, almonds, barley, and dark Grenache grape-based Cannonau wine also make the list. And they do like their wine. The average islander drinks 8 to 12 ounces a day spread throughout the day. They bust out this high-test, polyphenol-laden red stuff for breakfast, lunch, *and* dinner. Hey, you would be drinking heavily, too, if you had to eat casu marzu all the time.

The most striking feature about the island's oldest residents is their extreme level of physical activity. The average 80+-year-old male Sard shepherd walks more than 5 miles every day on demanding terrain. Many live in vertical homes that require heavy climbing. Poulain and Pes drilled down into diet and activity and theorized that this improved cardiovascular fitness was the primary reason for their blue zone status. Although diet and exercise are crucial to their well-being, could there be something unique in the isolated gene pool of central Sardinia that promotes longer life?

Ironically, while Sardinia is now thought to be a shining example of modern longevity and well-being, it used to be considered a pretty unhealthy place. Malaria has been endemic there since it was introduced by North African workers during the Carthaginian invasion in 502 BC.[7] Even the word, *mal-aria,* is Italian for "bad air." Malaria worsened in the final years of the 19th century with 20,000 reported deaths. In a country known for its malarial outbreaks, Sardinia reigned supreme. The problem became so bad that in 1900 the government began issuing large amounts of free quinine, the *"Chinino di Stato."* In the 1920s and 1930s Mussolini's massive reclamation and drainage projects were rolled out to produce arable farmland and attack the natural environment of the primary malaria vector, the anopheles mosquito. By the eve of World War II, malaria seemed to be under control.

When the war went sideways for the Fascists, political survival surpassed disease containment as the country's top social priority. In 1943, German troops intentionally flooded the southern plains along with the Pontine Marshes south of Rome to try to slow Allied progress through Italy. Thousands of bomb craters became convenient mosquito habitats. Malarial cases skyrocketed. Nearly everyone in Sardinia was exposed to the disease. By 1946, cases spiked to include 74,600 victims and 146 deaths, leading to the creation of the Rockefeller Foundation Sardinian Project.[8] This controversial experiment was designed to eradicate the disease by wiping out the parasite-carrying anopheles mosquito population. The Rockefeller Project (1946–1951) cost $12 million and used 32,000 workers to spread more than 267 metric tons of DDT throughout an island the size of New Hampshire. Ultimately, they failed to eliminate the anopheles, but still succeeded in eradicating malaria on Sardinia.

What does malaria have to do with Sardinian longevity? Maybe nothing. Maybe it's just a cool public health story about how this Italian island saved the swamps of post-war Long Island and New Jersey from becoming experimental targets of government-funded clouds of DDT. Maybe it is something more. Scientists now believe that endemic malaria in the Sardinian environment selected for people resistant to the disease. This is an important point because malaria is a ruthless killer that creates tremendous evolutionary pressure. Children die young, and individuals with protective genetic mutations gain a huge survival advantage. Although comprehensive genetic analysis of Sardinians has not yielded any unique cardiovascular or cancer-fighting mechanisms, a malarial-fighting genetic mutation called TNFSF13B has been discovered.[9] This gene produces a protein called B-cell activating factor (BAFF). More BAFF means more immunologically active B cells to curb-stomp the parasitic Plasmodia that cause malaria.

Genetic victory against malaria exacted a heavy toll. Like many cellular mutations that confer resistance against potentially lethal infections, including sickle-cell trait (malaria) and herpes (bubonic plague), TNFSF13B

**WHAT DO ALL BLUE ZONES HAVE IN COMMON?**

Older people are very active and tightly integrated into the community (they also regularly drink alcohol). Opa!

demands a dangerous pact with the body. Unleashing an army of infection-fighting B cells inevitably leads to collateral autoimmune damage to host nerves and tissues. As a result, Sardinians live a long time but have the world's highest incidence of multiple sclerosis, lupus, and many other disabling autoimmune diseases.

Maybe anti-aging DNA hacks aren't the answer. If there is no genetic gold here, then what's the real Sardinian century secret? Hopefully, it's all that wine and exercise, but not that awful casu marzu.

## FROM DEATH TO LIFE

Walking the idyllic beaches of coral-rimmed Okinawa today, it's hard to imagine this was the site of some of the fiercest fighting in World War II. More than 300,000 people perished on this remote, typhoon-beaten Pacific atoll in the final years of the war. Half of the dead were civilians caught up in the horror, destruction, and atrocities of the bitter conflict. In 1949, *Life* magazine described Okinawa as "an ugly, cluttered graveyard of rotting material left over from the Pacific war, a place garrisoned by depressed and sullen troops and populated by 600,000 hopeless natives."[10] Ironically, important lessons about healthy living have risen out of the haze and rubble of war.

Because of its strategic importance, the archipelago remained under the control of the US military until it was finally returned to Japanese rule in 1972. At the time, the local public health system of this economically poor island was in disarray. Efforts to improve rural health in the region led to a detailed study of the prefecture's population demographics by the country's Ministry of Health and a surprising discovery. Okinawans are old. I mean, like really, really old. Now in its 36th year, the Okinawa Centenarian Study, founded by Tokyo cardiologist Makoto Suzuki and later joined by Canadian researchers (and twins) Bradley and Craig Willcox, found that locals over 65 were some of the oldest people in the world.[11, 12, 13] With an average life expectancy of more than 89 years, Okinawans lived more than 10 years longer than people in the rest of the world. For example, in Okinawa, 6.5 people per 10,000 live to be 100, compared to only 1.73 per 10,000 in the United States. More importantly, Okinawa was the healthiest prefecture in Japan, with 80 percent fewer heart attacks than in the United States, little or no obesity, little or no dementia, and very few cases of stroke or cancer.

Why Okinawa? The poorest and most remote of all Japanese regions, it would not appear to be an obvious pied-à-terre for healthy aging. Populated for at least 32,000 years, the islands were once the independent kingdom of Ryukyu and were traditionally considered to be a place of extended life.[14] The Chinese called it the land of the immortals, a reference to the Taoist belief in *Penglai,* a Shangri La-like island where eternal life was possible. After it was forcibly annexed by Japan in 1879, the islands became riddled by a century of fighting, famine, and poverty. Okinawans were forced to adapt to their circumstances with cruel efficiency and effort just to survive.

Older Okinawans eat a severely calorie-restricted diet high in complex carbohydrates and limited in protein. Many still start their meals with the Confucian reminder, *Hara hachi bu,* to eat only until they are 80 percent full. Prior to WWII, more than 60 percent of their diet consisted of the imo, a purple Okinawa sweet potato, soybeans, mugwort tea, brown rice, turmeric, and a bitter melon called goya. The imo contains the powerful antioxidant sporamin. Turmeric is closely related to ginger and contains the anti-inflammatory chemical curcumin, which may slow dementia. Goya seems to have anti-diabetic effects. While there is some meat in the traditional diet, they prefer a fat-skimmed pork that is stewed for days until it is mostly just a slurry of protein and collagen. Damn, even my mother wouldn't have done that to a braciola. They also dig the seaweed kombu and wakame, both rich in micronutrients such as carotenoids, folate, magnesium, iron, calcium, and iodine.

Whatever longevity advantage they have on their island they lose as soon as they leave Okinawa. The most likely reason for this is that when they leave Okinawa, they switch from a spartan, calorie-restricted, plant-based diet to a calorie-heavy Western diet loaded with processed food. Early genetic mapping of super elderly Okinawans indicates that they may have some favorable insulin and metabolic epigenetic clusters that could be triggered by caloric restriction.[15] We'll go over how calorie restriction works to help you live longer later on in Chapter 4, The 4-Hour Rule.

## NEVER REGRET THY FALL[16]

Ikaria is unique. The enigmatic Greek island juts steeply out of the northern Aegean Sea 30 miles off the coast of Turkey. It was once connected by the same mountain range with Samos and Asia Minor. Many historians believe it is named for Icarus, who plunged to his death in a pile of melted wax and feathers in its waters after he and his father, Daedalus, escaped Minoan Crete. Greco-Roman mythology holds that Zeus's son, Dionysus, the god of wine, fertility, and ritual madness, was born on Mount Pramnos in Ikaria. Although inhabited since the Neolithic period, the island's inhospitable terrain, dangerous waters, and lack of natural ports kept it isolated from the rest of the Aegean throughout antiquity.

Despite these physical barriers, millennia of war, famine, poverty, and natural disasters gradually scarred and depopulated Ikaria. Carian pirates, Ionians, Phoenicians, Athenians, Spartans, and Persians invaded, pillaged, and gradually deforested the island. Despite a brief period of prosperity during the 5th century BC when the island population peaked at 13,000 under Athenian control, the Peloponnesian War with Sparta drove most people off the island.[17] Eventually, the Roman Empire converted Ikaria into an expensive penal colony for exiled senators and aristocrats. When the Roman Empire crumbled, Ikaria fell first to pirates, then Macedonia, then Samos, then Venice, then Genoa, and finally to the Ottoman Empire. The rebellious Ikarians finally broke away from the Turks in 1912, and were briefly independent before they were quickly annexed by the Kingdom of Greece. Unfortunately, a half-century of conflict and occupation followed. Two world wars and the bloody Greek civil war created widespread famine.

Starvation claimed 20 percent of the population. The island became known as the Red Rock after 13,000 communists were exiled there after the civil war between 1946 and 1950. It was not until the 1960s that the local economy began to recover when the Greek government began investing in infrastructure and tourism. Today the island has a population of 8,400 people.

Despite this strife, or perhaps because of it, the olive tree–dotted island has bred a sturdy population. In 1666, the Greek Orthodox bishop of Samos, Joseph Georgirenes, wrote, "The most commendable thing about this island is their air and water, both so healthful, that the people are very long liv'd, it being a very ordinary thing to see persons of a 100 year age, which is a great wonder, considering how hardily they live."[18] Since the times of Athenian rule, Ikaria has been known for its therapeutic hot springs. The baths contain a high percentage of minerals—and radioactivity. Say what? You heard me. Radioactivity, baby. Good old rads. The granite releases large amounts of radon isotopes into the groundwater that feeds the springs. It is ironic to think that while we spend millions of dollars in the United States trying to mitigate microcuries of radon to sell our houses, the Greeks are splashing around in their expensive, Geiger-busting mineral swill without apparent ill effect. They seem to prefer the thermal springs with higher radiation counts. Go figure.

The people of modern Ikaria continue to live longer and better than most of the world. A demographic study from the University of Athens pooled 671 locals over the age of 65 for detailed demographic analysis.[19] The study found that Ikarians are 2.5 times more likely to reach 90 than most Americans and 10 times more likely than Europeans. Even more provocative was that Ikarian men are more than four times more likely to make 90 than American men. And when they do make 90, the Ikarians absolutely rock it. They are three times more likely to be active than other Europeans and have dramatically lower rates of depression and 75 percent less dementia. Amazingly, 80 percent of men between 65 and 100 were still sexually active.

Elderly Ikarians are tough, hedonistic characters. They have survived decades of war, poverty, and famine. Many used to smoke, and most still stay up late, sleep late, and drink a lot. They are extremely active well into

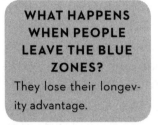

**WHAT HAPPENS WHEN PEOPLE LEAVE THE BLUE ZONES?**

They lose their longevity advantage.

their nineties and eat a lean diet loaded with fresh vegetables drenched in olive oil. Their traditional diet includes fish, red wine, potatoes, garbanzo beans, black-eyed peas, olives, sage, mint, lentils, and goat's milk. They also love eating dandelion weeds called *horta*. They eat these nasty turnpike weeds boiled, steamed, or in salads drenched in olive oil. There's not much meat in their diet, and they go easy on the sugar. We eat about a half a pound of meat a day in the United States, but Ikarians eat meat only once a week. Most (87 percent) drink a lot of ridiculously strong Greek coffee and herbal tea high in polyphenols and antioxidants.

Want to kick it, Greek-style? Eat some fish sprinkled with horta and olive oil. Hang out with friends. Drink some more wine. Have sex. Take a nap. Then throw back a cup of high-test joe. Repeat, repeat, repeat. Honestly, who cares if you reach 100, it already sounds like the perfect life. I told you it was a unique place.

## GERIASSIC PARK

Born from the collision of tectonic plates during the Pliocene epoch 3 million years ago, the Peninsula of Nicoya extends out from the northwestern corner of Costa Rica bordered by the Pacific Ocean on the west and the Gulf of Nicoya on the right. Its inhabitants, long known for their unusual longevity, remain isolated from the rest of Costa Rica by thick tropical forests and rugged mountain ridges, some as high as 3,000 feet. Its starkly beautiful, biodiverse environment and waterfalls have crafted a kind of geriatric Jurassic Park. Even in 1904, Swiss geographer Henri Pittier remarked that "in no other place are people blessed with such long lives."[20]

The region's natives descend from pre-Colombian Chorotega Indians. Nicoya is named for the chief of the Chorotega when the Spanish conquistadors arrived in 1523. The Chorotega were the most advanced of the indigenous Costa Ricans at the time. They spoke Mangue, a language that they brought with them from their original home in central Mexico's Cholula Valley. After the conquest by Spain, the Nicoya Peninsula struggled with poverty and disease. It was seceded to the Nicaraguan State of Leon in 1787. Following the liberation of Central America by the 1815 Mexican War of Independence, political chaos ensued. The Nicoya Peninsula along with much of northwestern Costa Rica was initially considered a province of newly formed Nicaragua in 1821. However, by 1824 the region voted for secession and joined Costa Rica.

Modern Costa Rica has a population of 4.5 million and is the second most densely populated country in Central America, after El Salvador. Nicoya is different. Its remote pristine beaches draw increasing numbers of tourists, but it remains a rugged and geographically isolated place. Much of the peninsula is still accessible only by air, bridge, or ferry. If you want to get around the peninsula, you better know how to handle an ATV.

Starting in 2008, Luis Rosero-Bixby from the University of Costa Rica performed a detailed demographic study of Costa Ricans and found they had a 14 percent lower mortality rate than other developed countries.[21] Costa Rican men older than 90 live 6 months longer than similar men in any country in the world. Not bad, but not enough to stamp my passport for. All that changed when Rosero-Bixby analyzed the Nicoyan data.[22] He discovered that men in the remote region outlived everyone in the world. A 60-year-old Nicoyan male has a seven times greater chance of reaching 100 than a Japanese male and lives an average of 2.2 years longer. Mysteriously, Nicoyan women do not share this survival advantage. Even more intriguing was the finding that when Nicoyans moved away from the peninsula, they lost their longevity edge.

What is it about Nicoya that helps its inhabitants live longer? Aging is a complex process that is driven by alteration to our chromatin, which includes DNA and the histone proteins that package and control our genes. The study of how genes are manipulated by these histones is called epigenetics. Human studies have found two genetic biomarkers of relative biological aging and stress: telomere length and DNA methylation rate. Telomeres are repetitive protective DNA sequences on the tips of chromosomes that gradually unravel and shorten during every mitotic division. A Stanford University study led by David Rehkopf found that Nicoyans older than 60 had notably longer telomeres than other Costa Ricans.[23] Good, right? Maybe.

DNA methylation is an epigenetic process driven by environmental changes that cause covalent bonding of methyl groups to cytosine to the 5' carbon of cytosine nucleotides, usually at cytosine-phosphate-guanine dinucleotide groups (CpG). Methylations can change the amount and types of proteins coded by the DNA. Basically, they mess with the body's motherboard. Higher methylation rates have been associated with aging and stress. It can also cause gradual mitochondrial damage that can cause sarcopenia (muscle atrophy) and the frailty of old age. In another study of elderly Nicoyan white cell DNA, Rehkopf's group discovered they had a 7.9 percent lower rate of CpG methylations than other Costa Ricans.[24] This suggests that a generally healthier, younger immune system may be one of their main longevity advantages.

What is it that has caused these epigenetic changes? Nicoyans differ from other blue zoners in that they eat a prosaic plains diet that includes meat, chicken, beans, and rice. Okay, it has a low glycemic index and is high in fiber, but the diet isn't really that special. They don't drink much milk, instead getting calcium and magnesium in large supply from the locally hard water and the lime they add to their tortillas. They are a very physical people who stay active and work well past age 90. Exercise might be one of the keys. Their telomere length advantage of 81 base pairs is similar in scale to that seen in people who hit the gym daily.

Could there be something in the air or land of the peninsula that helps them live longer? Doubtful. Costa Rica's dirty little secret is that it is the highest consumer of pesticides per square acre in the entire world. The whole damned world. Between 1977 and 2006, they imported 184,817 metric tons of pesticides and had a 340 percent increase in use.[25] We're talking the big guns here: paraquat, diquat, mancozeb, chlorothalonil, etc. These guys are the darlings of Monsanto. Incredibly, they don't even handle the stuff safely. Costa Rica averages about 2,000 pesticide poisonings every year.[26]

Add to that widespread exposure to industrial pollutants like chromium, benzene, and diesel exhaust, and Costa Rica's *pura vida* starts looking well, less *pura*. One interesting point is that paraquat is known to cause increased mitochondrial stress and higher levels of potentially toxic intracellular concentrations of reactive oxygen species. I guess what doesn't kill you might really make you stronger. Either way, I'm starting to rethink my whole ex-pat *Tuck Everlasting* fantasy plan. Maybe we should be looking for longevity answers closer to home. Next.

## MY BLUE HEAVEN

If there is a place that shows that where you live is less important to living longer than how you live, it is the newest addition to the blue zone list: Loma Linda, California. Located 60 miles east of Los Angeles, Loma Linda (Spanish for beautiful hill) looks like any other southern Californian suburb. Except for all the old people. At its core is a community of 9,000 Seventh-Day Adventists, a religion that takes the teachings of the Bible seriously—and literally. They believe the body is an actual temple of the Holy Spirit. What does that mean? No smoking, no drinking. Half of them do not eat meat. Exercise is encouraged, and the community is focused on the church and the medical center.

Longevity data has been flowing from this enclave for more than a quarter of a century and is finally taking hold. Adventists simply live longer. The average SDA male lives 7.3 years longer than the average Californian male, and SDA women live 4.4 years longer than other Californian women.[27] When you look at vegetarian Adventists, the differences are even more striking. Vegetarian Californian SDA males live 9.5 years longer than average non-veggie Californian men. Vegetarian Californian SDA females live 6.1 years longer than average non-veggie Cali girls. Impressive.

When it comes to diet, the SDA data suggests that how much you eat may be as important as what you eat. The biggest difference between vegetarian SDA folks and their meat-eating comrades was weight. The egg-eating vegetarians tipped the scales at 16 pounds lighter than the carnivores. Strict

30#

vegetarians averaged 30 pounds lighter. This translated to significantly less cardiovascular disease and diabetes.[28] The Adventist Church, like the Greek Orthodox, also emphasizes fasting periods, which may contribute to the general lack of obesity in the community. The grass may be leaner on the greener side of the street.

Vegetarian SDA men seem to also have some other things meat-eaters don't. Bad sperm. Researchers at Loma Linda University Medical School found that vegetarian SDA men have sperm counts that are one-third *less* than meat eaters.[29] What sperm they did have were lousy swimmers; only 33 percent were active, and very few were hyperactive. The 4-year study concluded that this compromised fertility might be the result of suppressive phytoestrogens in soy products, vitamin deficiencies, or residual pesticides in diets heavy in fruits and vegetables.

And then there is the matter of breakfast. Turns out Will Keith Kellogg and his brother John Harvey Kellogg were hard-core SDAs. They started out running a health resort in Michigan called the Battle Creek Sanitarium, based on SDA principles. In 1906, after years of doling out diet reform and enemas, they formed the Battle Creek Toasted Corn Flake Company, which became the Kellogg Company in 1922. A hundred years of breakfast propaganda have followed. That's not that grrrrrreat.

∞

For the moment, the blue zones continue to offer more questions about aging than answers. But there are some lessons here. Humans are a tough species. Difficult environments and stress seem to select for the strongest among us. Take those hardy genetic ingredients and blend them with daily exercise, a sensible plant-based diet, sex, work, and a strong sense of community, and you probably have the recipe for tacking on a solid 10 bonus years of good living. For now, many of the genetic secrets of longevity remain hidden in the dark, unknown stretches of our DNA. Whether or not you were born with hardy genes, the lessons we've learned from the blue zones can still give you a serious edge on aging.

The story of meaningful longevity is less about *where* you live and much more about *how* you live. We are a tough breed, us humans. Our bodies are machines built for heavy use. Our main evolutionary advantages are our resourcefulness and our metabolic flexibility. Our systems thrive on a little stress and respond to challenge. To really understand what you need to do to live longer, feel younger, and be more energetic, you're going to have to get serious about learning how your body really works. Now let's roll up those sleeves, folks, and prepare to get a little dirty. We're entering the crucible.

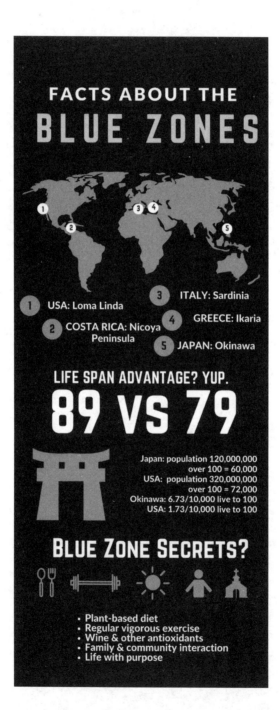

# FACTS ABOUT THE
# BLUE ZONES

1. USA: Loma Linda
2. COSTA RICA: Nicoya Peninsula
3. ITALY: Sardinia
4. GREECE: Ikaria
5. JAPAN: Okinawa

## LIFE SPAN ADVANTAGE? YUP.

# 89 VS 79

Japan: population 120,000,000
over 100 = 60,000
USA: population 320,000,000
over 100 = 72,000
Okinawa: 6.73/10,000 live to 100
USA: 1.73/10,000 live to 100

## BLUE ZONE SECRETS?

- Plant-based diet
- Regular vigorous exercise
- Wine & other antioxidants
- Family & community interaction
- Life with purpose

# 2

# THE CRUCIBLE

"Life is a complex, profound, and fluid dialogue between the genome and the environment."
—CARLOS LÓPEZ-OTÍN, 2016

IN MANY WAYS, SCOTT and Mark Kelly are a lot like me. We lived in the same town in New Jersey. We went to the same high school. Like most kids, we dreamed big. Epic, expansive adventures full of mountains, jungles, oceans, planets, and stars filled our future. We wanted to explore, adventure, and discover. We wanted to be astronauts. The difference between us is that the Kelly brothers lived those dreams. They became accomplished Navy fighter pilots and joined the US space program in 1996. They were part of a crucial NASA initiative to assess the possible toxic effects of outer space on the human body, the NASA Twins Study.[1] While the project was planned to learn more about life in space, it turns out that it may hold the key to living longer here on Earth (Figure 1).

Scott spent 1 year on the International Space Station (ISS) while his identical twin, Mark, remained earthbound. NASA scientists performed an extensive array of tests on the brothers before, during, and after Scott's year

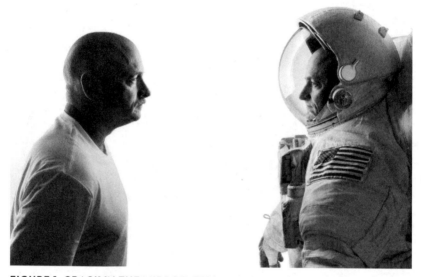

**FIGURE 1: CRACK IN THE MIRROR.** DNA sequencing and RNA analysis of astronaut twins Mark and Scott Kelly (Scott's on the right) reveal the powerful effects of environment on our genomic profile. (*Photo courtesy NASA.gov*)

in space, including a thorough analysis of the brothers' genetic profiles. The unexpected early results of those tests have now been released and can be described in one word. *Change*. When Scott first returned from orbit, he was 2 inches taller than Mark. Why? Without the constant downward pull of gravity, his vertebral disks had swollen. Despite vigorous exercise in zero gravity, he also lost calcium and bone mass. But the biggest surprise was found in how Scott's DNA, his genetic blueprint, had changed and diverged from his twin. Most astrobiologists believed that the constant bombardment of high levels of cosmic rays (10 times more than Earth) and the caloric constraints of life aboard the ISS would permanently damage his DNA and leave Scott at high risk for cancer, organ failure, and early death. They were wrong. Life in space did change Scott's DNA, but in different and unexpected ways.

As we've discussed, telomeres are long, repetitive sequences of DNA that protect our chromosomes from harm during cellular division.[2] When the telomeres get long, a protein called TZAP binds to them, and the repeated sequences are trimmed off. Normally, every time a cell rips open and divides as we age, a little more telomeric length is lost. Like a burning fuse leading to a catastrophic end, these canonical DNA sequences gradually fray and dissolve. When the telomeres are finally exhausted, cellular division stops and the coding portions of the chromosome unwind. The cell dies. Called the Hayflick Limit after Dr. Leonard Hayflick, the biologist who first discovered it, telomeric erosion was thought to be an irreversible, ultimately fatal process. The equation was simple: Longer telomeres equaled longer life. Only cancer cells possessing an enzyme called telomerase, which prevented their attrition, were thought to be immortal.

NASA prepared for the worst. They fully expected the cosmic rays and stresses of space to completely fry astronaut DNA. NASA believed deep space missions would be doomed by this fatal flaw. But space failed to corrupt Scott's telomeres. In fact, they became *longer* after he left Earth. Even more surprising was that when he returned home, his newly augmented telomeric DNA rapidly wore away back to the length of his brother Mark's earthbound chromosomes. The response of telomeres to stress is much more complicated than first thought and involves a symphony of TERT proteins that interact with telomerases to maintain an optimal length. In fact, telomeric length may have a "Goldilocks zone." Too short and the DNA unravels, leading to cell death. Too long and certain cancers accelerate.[3]

The genomic sequencers revealed even more unsettling data for NASA. To pack all our genetic data into our tiny nuclei, the body uses proteins called histones to fold, kink, and twist the DNA into tight packets. Nearby genes along these intricately twisting chromosomal limbs begin to interact with one other to determine which ones will be turned on or off. Every protein, cell, and organ we make and maintain is driven by this constantly changing pattern of gene expression. Yup, I'm talking epigenetics. As we age, our DNA and the cladding proteins that manage these genetic ladders are always changing and evolving. Environmental stresses lead to methylations that fundamentally change our genetic profile as we age. These gene mods lead to changes in the way that we produce proteins. Another term for this translation and production pipeline is *gene expression*.

Most scientists expected Scott's space-ravaged DNA to show dramatically more methylation than his brother's. They were wrong again. His DNA had far *fewer* methylation changes than his brother's. Had orbital spaceflight made Scott's cells chemically younger? Was there a phantom space immortal gene that was activated by all that height and distance? Hold on folks, I know what you're thinking. Before you sign up for a trip to Mars on the USS Ponce de Leon, you should also know that Scott's space-acquired DNA changes led to more than 200,000 changes in his RNA, drastically altering his protein production pipeline. Most of these changes remain unidentified. But the most surprising thing about the cellular changes that Scott experienced in space was just how quickly they reversed. One year after Scott returned to Earth, his DNA profile was once again nearly identical to his twin's. This confirms what many biologists have long suspected: Our DNA quickly and *reversibly* adapts in response to environmental demands.

Our body's genetic editors, ATP-dependent DNA binding and rearranging enzymes called helicases, are constantly marking and changing our genetic text. Mapping these chromatin edits creates a kind of epigenetic clock that gives researchers a way to comparatively study aging. Using this technique, a team from the University of California Los Angeles lead by Steven Horvath has found that cells deep in the brain's cerebellum age much more slowly than the rest of the body and identified the genes that might control this aging resistance.[4] Horvath and his colleagues have now joined hundreds of scientists around the world in the hunt for ways to snuff the genetic fuse and change the way we age.

To put it simply, our genetic blueprint can be modified. The implications of this are clear. We are not genetic prisoners. Our DNA is engaged in an active, dynamic dialogue with our environment. And nurture beats the crap out of nature. We are free to shape our future selves based on the lifestyle choices we make. All this freedom carries a terrible burden: the responsibility that how we eat, exercise, and interact with our physical and emotional environments fundamentally changes us from the inside out. And it very well may determine how much time we get. Now that you've been named CEO of You, Inc., it's time to walk the factory floor.

## RACE AGAINST THE MACHINE

The human body is a violent and wondrous instrument. It is the crucible of life. The heart beats more than 100,000 times a day with enough pressure to squirt a column of blood 30 feet in the air. Lungs with a 1,500-mile network of airways exchange toxic carbon dioxide for oxygen across a surface area the size of two tennis courts. Kidneys recycle more than 400 gallons of blood every day while releasing hormones that spur red cell production and activate vitamin D for bone health. The liver serves more than 500 different functions and controls glucose levels in the blood and energy storage in fat. The spleen acts as a massive transfer station, filtering and recycling worn-out blood cells and proteins. It also stores lymphocytes, establishing an ammunition depot for an early warning immune defense system.

Our senses are just as dynamic: Fingers so sensitive to imperfection they can perceive nanowrinkles. Ears that can detect pressure fluctuations of one billionth of an atmosphere. Eyes that see with the resolution of a 750 MB camera. A nose that can distinguish one trillion different scents and a tongue that can differentiate 50,000 tastes. The neural network that processes all this data is equally amazing. Nerve fibers transmit critical environmental data to the spinal cord and brain at speeds exceeding 170 miles per hour. A billion brain cells fit in a grain of sand, and each feed a trillion neural connections. Torrents of images are processed in milliseconds in the cerebellum, while memories stored deep in the recesses of the hippocampus are accessed faster than a supercomputer. The amygdala provides emotional resonance, fear, aggression, and social context. Acting like a wireless thermostat, the hypothalamus regulates body temperature, thirst, and hunger through hormonal control. The bottom line is that we don't use 10 percent of our brains. We use 100 percent. Every part of our brain is in play, driven by swirling hydroelectric clouds of thought. Bioelectric currents also drive wound healing and help the skeleton respond to dynamic gravity-driven stresses to maintain bone strength that rivals granite in compression.

Beneath this symphonic stage is an even more dynamic and complex microscopic world. Our bodies are made from more than 37 *trillion* cells organized into 250 different types.[5] Every second, millions of them die and are created in a biological tug of war where trillions of molecules are forged, circulated, and recycled. Ten billion cells are renewed every day. Every single day. Red cells race through 100,000 miles of vessels, lapping the entire body in less than a minute. These cellular drones pick up vital oxygen in the lungs and eject carbon dioxide waste as they pass through the crucibles of 300 million tiny pulmonary alveoli.

But there are barbarians at the gates of this empire. Our bodies host a microbiome of bacteria that dwarfs our own native cells by a power of 10. Many of these ancient intruders have turned allies, helping us digest food and process nutrients in the gut. But others are potentially lethal. Another crucial bit of early data from the NASA Twin Study demonstrated dramatic changes in the microbiome during spaceflight. The effects of this population shift remain unclear, but one thing that is certain is that not all the body's guest workers are friendly. War ravages this landscape. Bacterial and viral attacks are repelled and intruders are detained in daily combat with the environment. White cells attack and engulf bacterial invaders while lymphocytes fire from a defensive arsenal of more than two million immunologic proteins. Sentinel proteins identify, surround, and kill lethal mutant tumor cells. The pace of activity required to maintain the fragile balance of our superorganism is frenetic and drains precious energy resources. It is also ultimately unsustainable. Over time, our DNA accumulates damage, precious energy resources dwindle, our organs begin to fail, and we age. At least that's what we used to think.

**IT'S FULL OF STARS**

The human genome was first sequenced in 2001. It contains more than 3 billion constantly changing base pairs, but codes for only about 20,000 genes. The function of most of our DNA remains unknown.

In the past century, we have begun unlocking the secrets of aging. Initially, the discovery of the genetic code for life in a double-helical ladder of amino acids called deoxynucleic acid (DNA) seemed to offer a tidy explanation for how we lived, aged, and died. The code of life appeared to be a simple Scrabble game played with only four letters: A (adenine), T (thymine), G (guanine), and C (cytosine).[6] But when the human genome was finally sequenced in 2001, it became clear that only 2 percent of the genome codes for actual proteins. The purpose of the remaining 98 percent of DNA, much of it in long repetitive sequences, remains uncertain. We do know that the DNA is tightly coiled and kinked in an incredibly compact form in our chromosomes (Figure 2). Chromosomes are laced with a

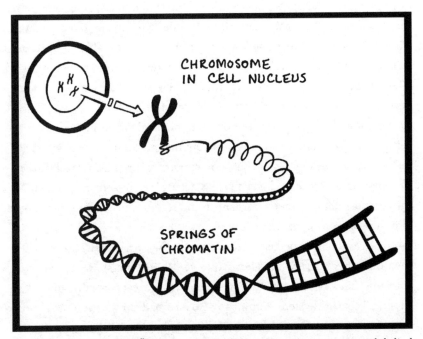

**FIGURE 2: PACKING THE PIÑATA.** Deoxyribonucleic acid (DNA) is a twisting triple helical ladder formed by nitrogen base-pairs rungs of adenine-thymine (AT) and cytosine-guanine (CG). A shell of cladding histone proteins kinks, bends, and squishes the DNA into chromosomes capped by protective telomeres. All this solenoid-shaped chromatin is stuffed into the cell nucleus like a tight little ball of microscopic Slinkies. (*Illustration: Jacob Scheyder*)

mutable protein shell that seems to protect and regulate our genes. Environmental stresses alter the shape and function of genes by chemically modifying cytosine molecules in our DNA through a process called methylation. As we saw with Scott Kelly, gene expression can be reversibly changed through this process.

Our DNA also dynamically responds to physical, emotional, and chemical stress. We grow differently based on how we interact with our environment on many levels. Scott and Mark Kelly, like all identical twins, developed unique tongue- and fingerprints due to the hydrostatic tidal eddies of their mother's womb. But some changes, including mutations, lead to indelible DNA modifications that are passed down through generations. For example, we know that about 8 percent of our DNA is alien. Not visitors from outer space, but emigres from *inner* space, spies who have injected thousands of bacterial and viral code sequences into our genome, while taking home bits of ours, during millennia of conflict. In fact, our unique blood types (A, B, AB, and O) are likely a direct result of these lateral gene swap meets.[7] Bacteria may be able to induce cancers in their host through this process of lateral gene transfer.

We know that 99.9 percent of our genome is identical in every human being, but what is it in the other 0.1 percent that makes us unique? What is it that makes one person age well but another poorly? How much is really driven by genetic inheritance, and how much is determined by our environment? Is the composition of our superorganism the real key, or is it our constantly morphing protein signature?

To be candid, if 10 percent of life relates to the genes you were born with, then the other 90 percent is how you live. We are not static. We are ever changing. This can be a good thing if you exercise, eat carefully, and have a supportive social system. But it can also be a bad thing if you make poor lifestyle choices. A very bad thing. For example, cigarette smoking leads to fundamental genetic changes that can last 30 years *after* you quit.[8] Thirty years. Still, many of the awful things we do to ourselves can be fixed with enough time and effort. Genetic redemption does await, but to make the right choices, you first need to know why. To do this, you need to look at your body as a factory—a beautiful, complicated organic machine that requires enormous amounts of energy to run. The hitch is that this busy industry of ours is not that efficient and we make mistakes. Lots of mistakes. We make errors copying our DNA, we make errors translating RNA, we make errors producing proteins, and we even screw up cleaning up all the messes that we created. Quality control is not our strong suit.

## ENERGY AND ERROR

Every time cellular division occurs, energy is expended. When errors happen, even more energy is drained. Tens of thousands of DNA copying mistakes occur daily and must be fixed. New research indicates that DNA replication is even more violent than we thought. DNA replication is not the rigidly ordered folding and packing we had been taught. Three-dimensional imaging of chromosomes during mitotic division reveals that they exhibit highly variable hyperkinetic bending, kinking, and twisting.[9]

We used to believe that after the DNA ladder is ripped open by helicases, the leading and lagging strands were copied in a coordinated and predictable fashion. Scientists have now learned from direct video of DNA replication that the process is far more chaotic. The leading and lagging strands are copied independently and at different speeds. This forces the helicases to have to constantly adjust the speed by as much as 80 percent to compensate. Yet another chance to screw up.[10]

**HOW MUCH DNA IS IN YOUR BODY?** If all your DNA were unwound, it would stretch over 10 *billion* miles. That's more than 100 times the distance between the Earth and Sun. The width of that incredible DNA string? Only 2 *nanometers!*

DNA's translation to RNA for protein production is another opportunity for molecular monkey business. The body produces trillions of proteins every minute, and the more we make, the more blanks we shoot. If the protein produced by the cell is misfolded or formed incorrectly, it will not work. Chaperone proteins called lysosomes help to refold the damaged protein or guide it to a cellular recycling area in a process called autophagy (Latin for "self-eating"). Rogue cancer cells must also be identified and assassinated to keep the organism alive. But there is a high price to pay for this vigilance. Every blunder worsens your body's deepening energy crisis. This titanic battle between energy and error forms the core of all our metabolic functions. It is what drives aging. It is a steel thread that is the key to extending life and health.

The foundation of metabolism is energy.[11] All living things produce energy like hydroelectric plants using free electrons to produce power. The unstable molecule, adenosine triphosphate (ATP), stores, moves, and releases these electrons like a rechargeable battery. To drive the metabolic production of ATP, both plants and animals need sugar (glucose) and break it down through a process called *cellular respiration* (Figure 3). Plants are much more sophisticated chemically than animals. They produce their own fuel using photosynthesis to charge their ATP batteries by combining light, water, and carbon dioxide in their chloroplasts.

Humans, like all animals, must *consume* our raw material in the form of proteins, fatty acids, complex sugars, and simple sugars to fuel our metabolic cycle. Our factories also need more energy and are much less efficient when faced with more complex fuel sources than simple ones. Why? Because everything must first be knocked down to the six carbon glucose molecules to even start ATP production. This energy pump also needs to be primed. You need energy to make energy. The body must use existing resources of ATP to break food down to glucose and then again to cleave each glucose molecule into two smaller molecules called pyruvic acid. The process of breaking down glucose is called glycolysis, and it's similar in all living things. It is a 10-step process requiring several critical enzymes that results in two pyruvate molecules for every glucose molecule that enters the pipeline. It also kicks out hydrogen protons that are picked up by NAD+ molecules to jump-start the second step of cellular respiration, the electron transport chain.

Even though we're not as efficient energy factories as plants are, we do have an ace in the hole that our leafy friends don't: the humble mitochon-

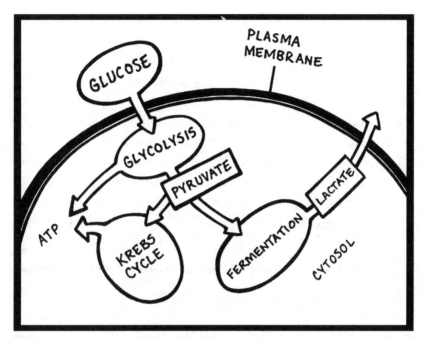

**FIGURE 3: THEY CALL ME MISTER KREBS.** Glucose passes through the cell's outer plasma membrane and gets broken down into pyruvate. When oxygen is present, it heads to the mitochondria, where the Krebs cycle uses NAD+ to move hydrogen protons (H+) down the electron transport chain and makes ATP+CO2+H2O (left). When oxygen is absent, pyruvate gets fermented in the cytosol to make a little ATP and recycle NADH back to NAD+. It's a beautiful thing. (Illustration: Jacob Scheyder)

dria. Like a factory within a factory, the mitochondria work like little powerhouses within our cells to make our ATP and move electrons around. These tiny organelles have their own cell membrane and their own DNA. Many scientists believe that mitochondria were once free-living single-cell organisms that invaded their animal hosts to set up symbiotic shop millions of years in the past. They gradually lost some of their own DNA as they continued to provide ATP "rent" for their hosts. When oxygen is present (aerobic), our bodies crank out most of our ATP molecules as the pyruvate is gradually broken down in the third, and busiest, stage of cellular respiration—oxidative phosphorylation (i.e., the Krebs cycle). Hydrogen molecules from the Krebs cycle flood across pumps in the mitochondrial membrane that release H+ proton to combine with NAD+ to ramp up the electron transport chain.

Like a churning hydroelectric plant, the elegantly beautiful enzyme ATP synthase converts the electrical energy created from this proton overflow into mechanical energy (Figure 4). This generates huge amounts of ATP that the body needs for its ravenous chemical energy demands. This chemical kiln runs reasonably efficiently, producing 30 to 38 ATP for every glucose molecule while producing only water, carbon dioxide, and some dissipated heat as waste. Leftover hydrogen protons are even carried off by NAD+ to make some bonus ATP in the electron transport chain. The bloodstream uses its red cells to absorb carbon dioxide and water waste

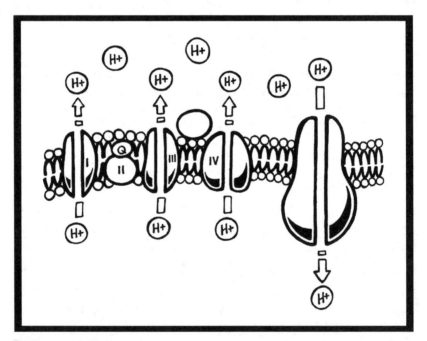

**FIGURE 4: PRIVATE HYDROELECTRIC PLANT.** Proton pumps (I-IV) embedded in the outer membrane of mitochondria squirt out H+ ferried over from the electron transport chain. Like a spinning waterwheel, ATP synthase (right) uses the rushing flow of H+ protons re-entering through its core to fuse ADP and free phosphate ions to crank out stored energy in the form of ATP. (*Illustration: Jacob Scheyder*)

from this cycle and haul it off to be dumped in the lungs. Now take a deep breath, then let it out. You've just experienced the Krebs cycle at work. One more deep breath and you will have cleared your mind for some more cool science stuff.

Our plant cousins conveniently use our leftover waste carbon dioxide to catalyze their own version of cellular respiration to make ATP. On the other hand, when there is not enough oxygen around, we must shift from using the Krebs cycle and convert to the far less efficient ATP production line of anaerobic respiration (fermentation). This pathway is used when muscles run out of local oxygen. It churns out a little ATP and produces lactic acid as a waste product, leading to muscle burning and cramps. Many people have the misconception that lactic acid buildup causes the muscle soreness that you get 2 or 3 days after a heavy workout. In fact, that soreness is driven by inflammation caused by local muscle damage. About a third of the lactic acid is shunted to the brain for use as an energy resource, and the rest is metabolized by the liver to make more pyruvate for glycolysis. Plants and yeast have a way better form of fermentation, producing ethanol and carbon dioxide as primary waste products instead of lactic acid. I want to personally thank the plant kingdom and my single-celled ancestor for the gifts of Bordeaux, baguettes, and breathing. *Vive la différence!*

## THE SEVEN PATHWAYS OF AGING

Over the last decade, new research has proven that the way we process and use metabolites and energy resources directly impacts how we age. The NASA Twins Study is a great example of how scientists use several indirect techniques to measure our biologic age, including telomere length, gene methylation (the epigenetic clock), and our changing RNA transcriptional signatures. Now we are learning more about the metabolic signs of aging. Biologist Carlos López-Otín and an international group of collaborators have narrowed these down to seven broad pathways of aging that all share a common theme: error. Let's take a closer look at each of these seven signs of cellular aging.

# 1. DNA DAMAGE

From the moment of conception, we devote ever-increasing energy resources to battle DNA damage. Life stresses the hell out of our genome. Solar rays, pollution, additives, chemicals, medications, and even diet shifts can trigger changes to our genetic code leading to metabolic disruption. In diseases that cause accelerated aging, like progeria, disabled genetic repair tools cause progressive metabolic failure and early death. Without functional nucleotide excision repair, DNA damage accelerates. Like a poorly wired motherboard, the metabolic system short-circuits and cascading nerve failure ensues. Cells with damaged DNA excrete interferon, which leads to early cellular senescence and kills stem cells. Nutrient sensing falls apart and insulin levels crash, leading to diabetes. An expanding wave of metabolic disruption widens, eventually knocking out glycolysis and the Krebs cycle in mitochondria. Normal tumor-monitoring proteins are shunted to try to control the mitochondrial failure but cannot keep pace. Hyperactive enzymatic activity driven by obesity and bacterial overload can further deplete cells of these tumor suppressors, causing chronic inflammation and cancer.

The hyperactivity of DNA repair enzymes like PARP1 creates even more demand on already depleted NAD+ resources in these patients, eventually shutting down NAD-dependent mitochondrial repair. Mitochondrial DNA damage and attrition are inevitable. Not a pretty picture. The good news is that some progeria patients respond well to interferon suppression and NAD+ precursor supplements that compensate for their genomic instability. The lessons learned from these unfortunate people highlight the complex connections between genetic alterations and metabolic activity.

# 2. ERODED TELOMERES

The shortening of telomeres presents somewhat of a dilemma for researchers. Is shortening one of the causes of aging or merely a result? Mice that lack telomerase, the enzyme that maintains telomere length, exhibit signs of accelerated aging with particularly poor mitochondrial production and development. Stem cells also show early exhaustion. Well, if too little telomerase is bad, then more must be good. Right? Maybe not. Cancer cells have 10 to 20 times the amount of telomerase of normal cells, leading to uncontrollable growth. Because of this, any attempt to enhance telomerase could end in malignancy or some screwed-up Deadpool thing.

We do know from animal studies that increased telomere shortening hurts the overall efficiency of the body's metabolic factory. Just like my dad's old Fleetwood, you need more gas in the tank to cover the same distance. Because of this, a diet higher in carbohydrates can help partially compensate for this lousy fuel efficiency. Can we slow down telomere attrition without resorting to potentially dangerous chemical mods? One new study suggests that daily exercise and decreased amounts of food force the body to be more efficient and decrease telomeric attrition. This is one possible reason why Scott Kelly's telomeres lengthened during his year in space.

## 3. EPIGENETIC ALTERATIONS

There is a strong link between enzymatic modifications of our chromosomes and changes in metabolism. The two main ways our genes are changed are through the enzymatic pathways of acetylation and methylation. The end effect is that we all develop a unique epigenetic footprint that determines how our metabolism is wired. Like a signature, some aspects are reversible, while others are not. A fascinating theory is that some of these environmentally driven changes in our genes may be inheritable. The existence of genetic memories could explain why obesity, diabetes, and other metabolic problems can be passed on to offspring after conception.[12, 13] Another mechanism could be the result of the enzymatic interaction between the mother and child during gestation and lactation.

Inflammation plays a central role in aging and may also be under epigenetic management. Adults seem to wind up either chronically inflamed or not.[14] This is determined by the activity of a specific inflammasome gene (IL-1 beta). Increased IL-1 beta activates platelets and neutrophils, leading to oxidative cellular stress, arterial stiffness, and hypertension. The environmental, dietary, and genetic triggers or suppressors of this inflammasome remain a mystery, but researchers believe caffeine may help block it. The important lesson here is that our genome is constantly morphing and adapting to our diet and environment.

## 4. LOSS OF PROTEOSTASIS

The shape and form of our proteins are critically important to how well they function. When they are misfolded or damaged, the body must first identify the malfunctioning proteins and then round up the suspects. A 2016 Nobel Prize was awarded to Yoshinori Ohsumi for his discovery of this process, called *autophagy*. Error demands energy. The body uses ATP-dependent sheepdog chaperone proteins to escort the culprits off to recycling areas in the cells called lysosomes where enzyme shredding occurs. When everything works well, we maintain a tight balance called proteostasis that allows real cellular renewal. However, as we age, the balance begins to slide and our garbage dump starts to overflow. This leads to system-wide metabolic stress and ultimately wrecks metabolism. Even worse, the sentinel monitoring system for tumor cells and infections declines. In contrast, healthy people who live past 100 usually have a robust proteosomal pipeline.

The failure of autophagy and loss of proteostasis may also cause Alzheimer's disease. In Alzheimer's, rogue tau proteins accumulate and gum up the entire protein recycling system, leading to dementia. Because the autophagic pathways are very enzyme dependent, they are a prime target for pharmaceutical intervention in the aging process. Metabolic changes can dramatically alter the natural process of apoptosis (programmed cell death) via levels of insulin-like growth factor-1 (IGF-1). When IGF-1 is low, precancerous cells are identified, killed, and disposed of with reasonable efficiency. As IGF-1 levels increase, this process becomes more porous, letting precancerous and damaged cells survive. Rising IGF-1 also gums up the autophagic recycling system and accelerates tau protein buildup in Alzheimer's. How  can you keep a lid on your IGF levels? A protein-regulated, plant-based diet has been shown to lower IGF-1 levels.[15] Intermittent fasting and time-restricted feeding also work. In contrast, high-protein diets stimulate IGF-1 production.

## 5. DEREGULATED NUTRIENT SENSING

The body is extremely sensitive to food and nutrient availability, responding within minutes with global metabolic changes. This occurs through a complex hormonal regulatory system that uses the proteins AMPK and sirtuins as a monitoring system. When we age, this sensory system dulls and screws up our metabolism in far-reaching ways. Remember our friend, the Krebs cycle? As nutrient sensing begins to decline, NAD+ supplies are depleted. This creates havoc throughout the body, slowing glycolysis and crashing ATP production. When glycolysis winds down, sirtuin and insulin production subside and we move carbohydrates into fat storage. This can lead to diabetes and obesity.

How can we fight this? If we take NAD+ precursor supplements like NR (nicotinamide riboside), the system can be overdriven to support efficient glycolysis. Exercise also helps boost your NAD+ levels. As we will see later, intermittent fasting and time-restricted eating (see Chapter 4: The 4-Hour Rule) work remarkably well to maintain efficient nutrient sensing and metabolic fitness.

The discovery of another nutritional pathway, the mechanistic target of rapamycin (mTOR) in 2009, may have even more profound effects on health and aging. When this complex metabolic pathway is suppressed in animal models, inflammation decreases, obesity resolves, insulin sensitivity improves, neurodegeneration slows, and autophagic recycling systems improve. Rapamycin, an antibiotic that torches mTOR, also kills cancer cells like Raid kills bugs. Too bad it also wipes out your immune system. Is mTOR the off-button for aging? We'll take a closer look at that in Chapter 16: Stranger Things.

## 6. MITOCHONDRIAL DYSFUNCTION

When NAD+ levels decrease with aging, the mitochondria begin to struggle with ATP production. Like factories trying to contend with dwindling resources, the mitochondria slow down and cellular functions decline. Because they produce energy by feeding their furnaces with oxygen, the mitochondria's unique DNA (mtDNA) is directly exposed to toxic free radicals in the cytoplasm. This naked mtDNA is damaged at a much higher rate than the host cell's own DNA that is sitting safely behind the secure walls of the nucleus. With less ATP around, the cellular energy crisis deepens, and mitochondrial DNA repair, cleanup, and the birth of new mitochondria (mitogenesis) shut down. Conversely, when NAD+ is plentiful, mitochondrial repair, turnover, and production are brisk. This leads to robust mitochondria, increased ATP production, and overall better system health and longevity.

## 7. CELLULAR SENESCENCE

Just like our bodies, each individual cell has a life span. The aging of individual cells is called cellular senescence. These dead and dying cells must be removed and broken down by the body to keep us healthy. If they are not reprocessed, cellular remnants lodge in tissue and cause harmful inflammation. An example of this is the way dead foam cells become trapped in the coronary arteries, leading to inflammatory-driven damage and heart disease. Treatments using senolytic medications will likely help the body deal with this problem. A recent Mayo Clinic drug study targeting p16 protein production, a marker seen in all senolytic cells, improved health and lengthened life span by 25 percent.[16] Some senolytic cells that escape detection have an even more sinister fate. They become cancers.

The central regulator of aging lies deep within the brain. In an animal model, scientists at Albert Einstein University have discovered a small group of neuronal stem cells in the hypothalamus that release exosomes full of microRNA messengers that fan out through the system to control the aging process through gene suppression and modulation.[17] Chronic inflammation in this zone can be fatal to these transcriptional lost boys. When they begin to die off, the pace of senescence quickens. Our metabolism begins to destabilize. DNA methylation changes build up, and shifts in the mRNA profile warp our protein signature. NAD+ levels crash to feed the escalating needs of faltering DNA repair crews. Wounds heal more slowly. Broken bones take longer to mend. Cell replacements become scarce. Intracellular communication falters. The result is that we begin a slow death spiral of scrambled metabolic function, failed insulin sensing, cumulative tissue damage, decreased energy, progressive inflammation, stem cell attrition, cognitive decline, and system-wide organ failure. Not the kind of golden years I had in mind.

What can we do? How do we escape this dark whirlpool? As it turns out, the metabolic connections that run through these seven routes of aging provide many ways to address the problems with aging and improve our lives. The science of metabolism gives us clear buoys to navigate the white water of aging. The beautiful thing is that most of these interventions require nothing more than a little knowledge, commitment, and discipline. The time to start living better and healthier is right now. No, no, no. No more foreplay. Let's get to work.

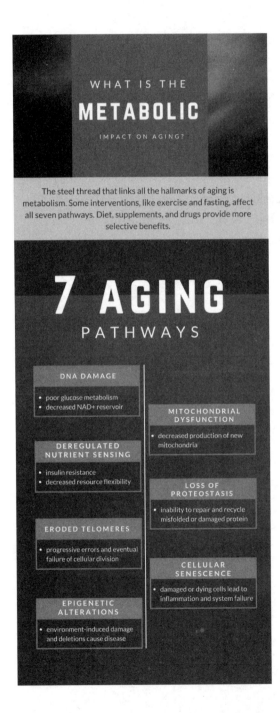

WHAT IS THE

# METABOLIC

IMPACT ON AGING?

The steel thread that links all the hallmarks of aging is metabolism. Some interventions, like exercise and fasting, affect all seven pathways. Diet, supplements, and drugs provide more selective benefits.

# 7 AGING
## PATHWAYS

**DNA DAMAGE**
- poor glucose metabolism
- decreased NAD+ reservoir

**MITOCHONDRIAL DYSFUNCTION**
- decreased production of new mitochondria

**DEREGULATED NUTRIENT SENSING**
- insulin resistance
- decreased resource flexibility

**LOSS OF PROTEOSTASIS**
- inability to repair and recycle misfolded or damaged protein

**ERODED TELOMERES**
- progressive errors and eventual failure of cellular division

**CELLULAR SENESCENCE**
- damaged or dying cells lead to inflammation and system failure

**EPIGENETIC ALTERATIONS**
- environment-induced damage and deletions cause disease

# 3

# ANCIENT INVADERS

"I am intimately involved, and obliged to do a great deal of essential work for my mitochondria . . . Each of them, by all accounts, makes only enough of its own materials to get along, and the rest must come from me. And I am the one who has to do the worrying."

—LEWIS THOMAS, *LIVES OF A CELL*, 1974

**MITOCHONDRIA ARE MISUNDERSTOOD. LIKE** their plant-locked chloroplast cousins, mitochondria have their own DNA, their own RNA, and their own protein-making ribosomes. Fundamentally, mitochondria and chloroplasts are the two most important structures to life on Earth. Chloroplasts, found exclusively in plants and algae, use carbon dioxide to make oxygen and energy, while mitochondria, found in animals, take oxygen and produce carbon dioxide and energy. The symmetry is inescapable. Since the discovery of mitochondria in 1881, the prevailing scientific belief has been that they were once free-living bacteria, caught and enslaved by ATP-starved eukaryotic masters in some endosymbiotic cataclysmic event more than 2 billion years ago. After all, the structure of mitochondria, marked by a labyrinth of inner folded membrane (cristae), is close to primitive bacteria. They are close in size (5 micrometers) and have no nucleus, their DNA is looped in a bizarre circle, and they can swim around their host cell freely. They produce ATP, the energy of life, and in return we provide room and board. Pretty straightforward deal, right?

Nothing could be further from the truth. Although mitochondria play a central role in energy production through oxidative metabolism, an expanding body of research indicates that they drive cellular communication and reproduction, telomeric stability, cellular growth, neurodegenerative disease, insulin sensitivity, obesity, cancer, inflammation, aging, and even death. This radical shift in perspective raises a simple question: Who is really running the show here? Are they parasites, symbiotes, or something very different? Careful genetic analysis now suggests that we have co-evolved with our mitochondria.[1] They have shifted much of their enzymatic heavy lifting to our cells, and we have yielded metabolic management duties to them. Even ATP production is now co-managed.

There are more than 1,500 different proteins at work in the mitochondria. While 13 important proteins needed for the electron transport chain and energy production are coded for by mitochondrial DNA (mtDNA), most of the proteins are coded for by the DNA in the nucleus and have to be folded up, packaged, and then shipped to the mitochondria to make the system work. Crossing the convoluted mitochondrial barrier and negotiating the internal maze of mitochondrial membranes is tricky business. To get this done, mitochondria use their own elaborate chaperone protein transport system. These tugboats check the quality of the incoming delivery and escort the proteins into the energy production pipeline. When the cell is injured or under stress, it delivers banged-up, unfolded proteins. This triggers an adaptive reaction from our mitochondrial overlords. The mitochondrial unfolded protein response (mtUPR) cranks up to try to deal with this problem. If the mtUPR is not overwhelmed, protein balance is maintained and the cell is forced to be more energetically responsible. Good boss. What happens when the mitochondrial proteins back up and start gumming up the cytoplasm? The cell is marked for death. Bad boss.

The mitochondria also match cellular and biological processes with the host nucleus through stretches of non-coding RNA. This synchronization may be one reason why mitochondria change shape, size, structure, and function in seconds to respond to stress or environmental challenges. They can also transfer bits and pieces of their DNA to other mitochondria or even migrate to another cell to find safe harbor. This communication may hold some secrets to longevity. Variations in mitochondrial proteins have been associated with increased life span in Japan. BTW, mtDNA is only inherited maternally during reproduction. Any mtDNA contributed by Dad is targeted and destroyed when sperm and egg fuse. Sorry, no boys allowed.

## FISSION AND FUSION

It makes sense that mitochondria are present in highest concentration where they are needed most for energy production: the brain and heart. Each has thousands of mitochondria per cell, while most muscles have only a few hundred and platelets have even fewer. Red cells, the stripped-down drones of the body, whose only job is to transport oxygen and dump off carbon dioxide waste, lack a nucleus and have no mitochondria. Mitochondrial replication is called fission, and it's key to maintaining high population density in critical zones. Scientists once thought this was a random and disorderly event but now believe it is carefully triggered. Unlike typical eukaryotic cells, mitochondria are devoid of a nucleus, and thousands of their small, naked circular chromosomes are sprinkled throughout the many baffles of cristae in the matrix.

A study at the University of California studying mitochondrial fission found that the contact points between the inner membrane fold and the outer membrane create a lasso around the mitochondrion.[2] In zones of mtDNA replication, called nucleoids, the protein noose around the mitochondrion tightens around until the barbell is pinched off into two distinct organelles. This guillotine style of chromosomal distribution is more loosely regulated than traditional cellular mitosis and might be a reason why mtDNA transfer errors occur. It also appears that we provide the proteins (dynamins) needed for our strange friends to pull this off. No wonder the quality control is so bad.

Damage to mtDNA can occur before, during, or after fission. Mutation rates in mtDNA are 50 times higher than in our nucleus-protected chromosomes.

This is because mtDNA is directly exposed to high concentrations of reactive oxygen species (ROS) and caustic nitrogen waste produced during ATP production. Luckily, mitochondria are a promiscuous lot with no sense of personal space. I know, you're shocked. When one mitochondrion gets in trouble, it can undergo cellular fusion. This occurs when adjacent mitochondria link membranes, blend proteins, and then mix their mtDNA. Although they are usually depicted as lima bean–shaped, mitochondria can go freestyle and take on long, filamented forms. Because they like to be close to one another, outer membrane contact is common via fingerlike dendrites. This allows communication and dynamic networking. When mtDNA damage is detected in one mitochondrion by another, fusion ensues and any extra leftover chromosomal material or damaged proteins after repair are jettisoned or trigger further fusion and fission cycles.[3] In a sense, they can hack their own genome.

Mitochondrial dysfunction due to ROS has also been linked to neurodegenerative diseases like Alzheimer's and Parkinsons.[4, 5] More than 24 million people have Alzheimer's. It results from toxic amyloid beta plaques that build up outside the neurons. The pathology is likely related to damaged recycling autophagic systems but is intimately linked to mitochondrial dysfunction. A whirlpool of ROS damage ensues that feeds amyloid accumulation, which then viciously leads to more damage. The amyloid binds to mitochondrial enzymes, which wrecks oxidative phosphorylation and ATP production, starving the brain. In Parkinson's, a similar but even more insidious process unfolds where alpha synuclein (Lewy bodies) and tau deposits form *inside* the neurons. When IGF-1 increases, the protective effects of apoptosis are lost and the autophagic system begins to collapse, eventually disabling even basic cellular protein transport.

As we have learned, however, DNA repair is an expensive proposition for the body, and energy depletion can be catastrophic. Compounding the problem is that the mtDNA repair system is not as robust as our own. To control the amount of damaging ROS produced during ATP production, mitochondria have evolved elaborate antioxidant defense mechanisms including glutathione, the pentose shunt system, and superoxide dismutase. They have also developed the ability to regulate the production of the ROS through a negative feedback loop. Even isolated mitochondria can detect buildup of the free radical, superoxide, by monitoring its final conversion product, hydrogen peroxide ($H_2O_2$), as it flows across their membrane gates. If antioxidant reserves have been overwhelmed, rising hydrogen peroxide levels can still tip off the mitochondria to scale back ATP production to drop ROS back to safe levels.[6] This may be why there is no China Syndrome–like reactor meltdown after heavy aerobic work.

Given the exposure of mtDNA to oxidative wreckage, mutation, and translational mayhem during fission, you can see why aging would first target those organs that have the highest concentrations of mitochondria— the brain, heart, and pancreas. Luckily, mitochondria are tough little guys and can take care of their own, blending DNA with their neighbors to help respond to stress damage. To understand how mitochondria control metabolism and health, we need to understand what happens when they age.

## THE MIDAS TOUCH

Oxidative phosphorylation occurs along the maze of inner membrane folds of mitochondria and accounts for 90 percent of all oxygen consumption in the body. Having lots of folded membranes may be awesome when you're using them to pump out hydrogen protons to make ATP, but they wind up causing problems in aging. The problem is that millions of cycles of membrane depolarizations gradually take a toll on the mitochondria. As we age, these membranes begin to leak like an old canvas tarp. This causes increasing release of $Ca^{++}$ with aging that blocks normal $K^+$ gate depolarization. An electric fence is created that stiffens the endothelial walls in the vascular system, blocking local nitric oxide flow and effectively choking off vital blood flow to organs and tissue. When you combine decreased vascular pliability, narrowed vessel dimeter from cholesterol plaques, and inflammation from senescent cellular debris, you have a recipe for a lethal heart attack.

Experimental models of mitochondrial dysfunction-associated senescence (MiDAS) have started to unlock how mitochondria control other aspects of aging and contribute to disease. Using cells with engineered mitochondrial dysfunction, Chris Willey and researchers at the Buck Institute for Aging devised an animal model for mitochondrial senescence that closely resembles aging in humans.[7] The MiDAS cells accumulate in fat and skin, leading to obesity, hair loss, and thin skin. The mechanism of MiDAS seems to be driven by decreased nicotinamide adenine dinucleotide (NAD+) to nicotinamide adenine dinucleotide hydrogen (NADH) ratios in the cytosol. In normal cellular respiration, mitochondria oxidize NADH to NAD+, using the H+ protons to drive ATP production by ATP synthase. In MiDAS, this system fails, NAD+ production crashes, and AMP and ADP levels soar. Bad things start happening. Metabolic failure activates the assassin protein, p53, which targets the cell for execution. Catastrophic MiDAS cell damage can be nearly fully corrected by restoring the correct NAD+ to NADH ratio. This has been done in the lab by adding pyruvate to suppress NADH processing or keeping the system charged up by simply adding extra NAD+. The MiDAS cell experiments strengthen the link between aging and metabolism and offer possible ways to safely steer it.

**HOW MUCH ATP DO WE NEED EVERY DAY?**

It's estimated that an active adult uses 1,000 ATP molecules every second. Over the course of a day we burn almost 70 kilograms of ATP!

## BREAKING NAD

Research has identified NAD+ as the key cellular factor in the control of metabolic enzymes including sirtuins (SIRTS), ADP-ribose transferases (ARTs), poly ADP-ribose polymerases (PARPs), and cyclic ADP-ribose synthases (CADPRs).[8, 9, 10] The MiDAS studies also demonstrate that NAD+ is key to slowing metabolic decline with aging.

Well that's great, but where can I get me some NAD+? There are several ways the body can make NAD+, but all of them dump NAD+ into one common reservoir for general metabolic withdrawal and use. We normally make most of our NAD+ through the nicotinamide salvage pathway. This is mediated by an important enzyme complex called NAMPT (nicotinamide phosphoribosyltransferase) that helps us capture and recycle most of the NAD+ we burn through each day. However, there are other, less efficient ways to get NAD+. Diet can be a source of NAD+. Niacin, a form of vitamin $B_3$, can be broken down in a three-step process called the Preiss-Handler pathway. But this will cost you some ATP. Good, but not great. The body can also break down the amino acid tryptophan to NAD+ using the kynurenine pathway. This is challenging and involves a lot of enzymatic steps. It can also lead to the development of immunologically tolerant cancer cells. Right, let's go back to salvage.

The salvage pathway is an intracellular process, and all the NAD+-consuming enzymes (SIRTS, ARTs, and PARPs) produce nicotinamide as a waste product. NAMPT uses all this nicotinamide and makes NAD+ and NMN. NAD+ levels rise with caloric restriction or exercise. NAD+ levels fall with high-fat diets and aging. The real problem is that the NAD+-producing salvage pathway begins to fail with aging. NAMPT levels drop in the brain, heart, pancreas, and skeletal muscle. This may be related to PARP1 exhaustion because of its role in repairing the accelerating DNA damage that accompanies aging.

There are seven sirtuin (SIRT) protein deacetylases that perform key metabolic functions throughout the body. The magnificent seven SIRTs fan out through the system to regulate metabolic functions. They are very sensitive to NAD+ levels and transduce energy signals via protein acetylation. These NAD+-dependent enzymes regulate protective biological functions by removing acetyl groups from key proteins. In all organisms ever tested, caloric restriction improves metabolic efficiency and can increase life span by 10 to 40 percent. The NAD+/SIRT pathway may increase longevity by activating a mitochondrial stress response that signals them to clean up the cellular mess. When protein acetylation of SIRT1 occurs, NAMPT levels rise and the salvage pathway gets cranking. SIRT1 helps manage our circadian clocks by deacetylating and changing some of the histones that kink and fold our chromosomes.[11] SIRT1 also deacetylates acetyl CoA, synthetase. This helps to regulate our circadian clock and provide metabolic efficiency.[12] Bottom line: more NAD+, more energy, more health = more life. Very cool.

SIRT6 regulates telomere stability and length along with inflammation. Loss of SIRT6 is found in progeria, where aging is rapidly accelerated. SIRT3 is the primary mitochondrial protein deacetylase and shoots up with fasting but declines with aging. SIRT3 is cool because it ramps up enzymes that shield our mitochondrial DNA, enable fatty acid production, improve oxidative phosphorylation, and suppress tumor development. If SIRT3 levels drop, a metabolic syndrome occurs resulting in diabetes, liver damage, obesity, hyperlipidemia, and vascular damage.

PARPs are like the enzymatic surgeons of the body—brilliant, self-absorbed, and expensive. PARP1 diagnoses DNA damage and determines whether to fix the error or just kill the cell. There are 17 genes alone that code for PARP-related proteins. These are the real deal, folks. In addition to performing DNA surgery, PARP1 powers ribosomal RNA creation and inflammatory control. Heavy PARP1 activity comes with a high energy bill and can quickly drain 80 percent of your *total* NAD+ reserves. Not counting the co-pay.

We also know that NAD+ is not just enzyme chow. It works its real magic when there's oxygen, moving electrons along the electron transport chain during oxidative phosphorylation to produce ATP. In the absence of oxygen, NAD+ shifts over to help produce whatever ATP it can in fermentation (along with lactic acid). The big problem is that all these metabolic processes compete for NAD+ from a single shared pool. As we get older, DNA damage accelerates and places increasing demands on NAD+-dependent repair systems like PARP. This exhausts NAD+ supplies and triggers SIRT1 shutdown. This sends a shudder through the entire metabolic system that causes even more DNA damage. An Icarian death spiral ensues as NAD+ demand exceeds supply.

It gets worse. Eat a high-fat diet and your NAD+ drops. Eat a high-protein diet and your NAD+ drops. Get older . . . and your NAD+ drops. The worst part about all this is that NAMPT, the one stupid enzyme needed for NAD+ salvage, is lowest where you need NAD+ the most—the brain, heart, pancreas, and skeletal muscle. NAD+ loss in the brain is devastating since it accelerates the formation of amyloid and tau deposits in Alzheimer's and Parkinson's. What happens when your autophagic recycling systems must put in overtime to deal with all that brain goo? That's right, NAD+ drops.[13, 14, 15] The downward NAD+ spiral tightens as circadian rhythms are disrupted by aging, further tangling the pipeline. Maintaining sufficient levels of intracellular NAD+ is critical to

**GAS GUZZLERS**
PARP1 enzymes can drain 80 percent of NAD+ supplies when repairing extensive DNA damage. Talk about a budget buster!

preserving the fragile truce between our nuclei and the mitochondrial hordes embedded in the cytoplasm.[16]

What can you do? We know that caloric restriction and exercise increase NAD+. Beyond that, the focus has pivoted to try to find ways to supplement the salvage pathway. Oral supplementation with nicotinamide riboside (NR), a form of vitamin $B_3$ found in small amounts naturally in milk, has been investigated to ramp up NAD+ supplies and correct the balky NAD+/NADH ratio that comes with aging. NR turns out to be readily bioavailable and is converted to NMN and then NAD+ along the latter stages of the salvage pathway. Studies in mice have shown that NR also activates mitochondrial repair systems including the unfolded protein response (UPR) that may be important in longevity. NR is now commercially available as an NAD+ precursor vitamin supplement. Although there is a dearth of human studies of NR, it has shown indirect signs of increasing NAD+ repletion and has been associated with only minor side effects such as headaches and flushing. In animals, the effects of NR supplementation are similar to calorie restriction and may be linked through mitochondrial metabolism.

NASA is also looking at ways to use NAD+ in overdrive to blunt the effects of cosmic rays in long-distance spaceflight. Scientists are testing nicotinamide mononucleotide (NMN) for this purpose as well as possible ways to feed the NAD+-dependent DNA repair system for patients undergoing high-dose radiation imaging or treatment. Still with me? Now you can ask. Yes, I do. I'm popping those NAD+ supplements like they are M&M's.

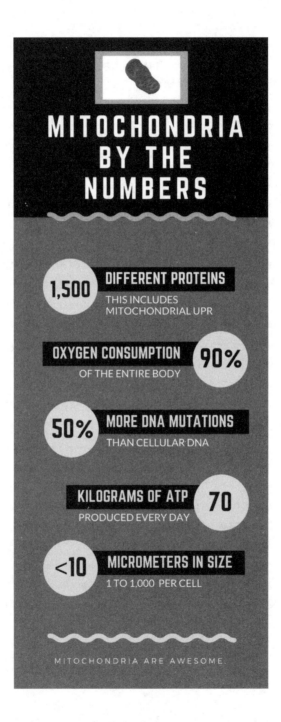

# 4

# THE 4-HOUR RULE

"I can think. I can wait. I can fast."

—HERMANN HESSE, *SIDDHARTHA*, 1922

**WHEN IS LESS, MORE?** Caloric restriction (CR) has been the only intervention that has been shown to maximize health and longevity in every species ever tested. The potential benefits of reducing caloric intake without causing malnutrition were first discovered by Clive McCay and his research team at Cornell University in 1935.[1] There was a prevailing belief at the time that increased metabolic rate was tied to decreased life span. If you could decrease metabolism, then you could live longer. McCay's early results on underfed rats were dramatic. The starving rodents lived 60 percent longer than their fluffier roommates. He reasoned that the fasting rats shifted into a conservation mode with slower metabolism that prolonged their lives. In the decades since, scientists have wrestled with the myths and mechanisms that underpin the profound, but sometimes unexpected, effects of caloric restriction and fasting.

While the potential health benefits of fasting were not investigated until the early 20th century, religions and ancient cultures have used it to treat disease for thousands of years. The Greeks used fasts to treat epileptic seizures.

> ## HOW DOES FASTING AFFECT METABOLISM?
>
> All forms of calorie restriction trick the body into mitochondrial energy efficiency, tumor growth suppression, and increased autophagic recycling.
>
> Your fat quickly rebels by sending uridine molecules to your brain to override the fasting order and force you to eat a bucket of delicious fried chicken. Don't fall for it.

Crazy? Not really. Brain activity is driven by neurons firing in response to chemical trigger proteins that cross tiny channels called synapses. With billions of neurons constantly working, the brain consumes an extraordinary amount of the body's energy supplies—up to 80 percent. This makes our nuggets extremely sensitive to metabolic changes.

Until recently, most scientists believed that fasting would result in decreased production of mitochondrial reactive oxidative species (mtROS), the potentially DNA-damaging by-products of energy production. They were wrong. In fact, the body's initial response to fasting is to increase mitochondrial oxygen consumption and ramp up oxidative phosphorylation. This leads to more mtROS. The failure of this to cause accelerated mitochondrial damage has called into question the traditional belief that mtROS are dangerous to the exposed DNA. How does increasing mtROS debris reduce seizure activity? The mtROS aren't just useless spent fuel cartridges hanging around to bang up our mtDNA. They also act like a neurologic volume control for the brain by tightly controlling the production of proteins that govern nerve firing. When levels of mtROS rise, two strong neuroinhibitors called GABA and serotonin increase. They raise the firing thresholds of the brain neurons, effectively quenching seizure activity. Hey, nobody said the Greeks weren't smart—after all, they did invent the screw.

## OF MICE AND MEN

What else does caloric restriction and fasting do? Lab studies suggest that their metabolic effects on the body are extensive and complex.[2] We've always thought that when food is scarce, our metabolism would slow down to conserve resources. Wrong. The first thing that happens is metabolic rates increase. The mitochondria immediately fire up the furnaces to provide more energy to you to go and get them some more food or to move to another place where food is more plentiful. For whatever evolutionary reason, this increase in oxidative phosphorylation starts burning through your NAD+ reservoirs. More oxidation means more energy in the form of ATP but also means more toxic reactive oxidative species (ROS) waste. Rising ROS stimulates a defensive increase in protective antioxidants. Sensing collateral oxidative mitochondrial DNA damage, PARP cleanup crews are dispatched and NAD+ levels plummet. Any cells not operating efficiently are chewed up for recycling. The body starts breaking down the staircases and burning the steps for fuel. The NAMPT salvage system gets moving to try to squeeze as much NAD+ out of the system as possible. To do this, the mitochondria are forced by rising SIRTs, the metabolic regulators, to be more metabolically "flexible." Remember the Krebs cycle? The mitochondria can use only glucose to make ATP without oxygen. When they are pushed to scavenging fat and protein to make energy, they burn through oxygen like crazy, forming even more ROS.

All this oxidative activity sends a shudder through the system. AMP-kinase (AMPK) levels start climbing, and this tells the mitochondria to start tightening their belts and divide. More mitochondria can temporarily produce energy if nutrients are available. Any NAD+ they do produce is used to keep the batteries charged up and the whole machine going until more food is found.

Maybe ROS production itself isn't the problem. Think about it: How can oxygen be that bad for us? Without it, we die. It is more plausible that ROS is a signal. Caloric restriction, when coupled properly to a functioning antioxidant system, works like a handshake. One of the most important enzymes in energy production, AMPK, senses ROS and NAD+ activity to adjust output. SIRT1 levels rise, spurring autophagy in the brain and other organs for recycling.[3] The SIRTs also get busy and start deacetylating stuff like PGC-1 alpha and FOXO transcription factors. New insulin-producing beta cells in the pancreas are generated to promote nutrient sensitivity. This may be one reason why type 2 diabetes responds so well to any type of caloric restriction. Any metabolic stressor is going to initially cause a rise in ROS and a compensatory spike in antioxidants, such as superoxide dismutase.[4] SIRT-1 also acts as a nutrient-dependent regulator of inflammation-triggering cortisol release.[5] This immunological jump start could explain why fasting can decrease inflammation, improve type 1 diabetes, and help fight infections.[6,7] Aging could be viewed as a breakdown of metabolic coupling that is reflected in decreased NAD+ supplies and NAD+-dependent receptor sensitivity. Maintaining a little oxidative stress in our lives is a good thing. It stimulates the liver cells to release hormones that trigger ketone production and fatty acid oxidation as it binds toxic IGF-1 to improve metabolism.[8] The message is clear: Eating less forces your metabolic system to work more efficiently. Although this doesn't necessarily mean you'll be thinner, it can help you live longer and healthier. Now if we could find a way to solve the whole hunger thing.

## PROPERTY OF STARDUST

One of the most important functions of the liver is to closely regulate blood sugar (glucose) levels. It also makes uridine, an RNA-building block that NASA believes may have originated from a wayward meteorite that crashed on Earth billions of years ago. Uridine is needed for RNA synthesis, glycogen production, and other crucial metabolic functions. This metabolic missing link binds our genetic code to protein production and energy regulation. When you are well fed, uridine sits around in the bile and is stored in the gallbladder. It then winds up in the GI tract, where it helps nutrients to be absorbed. This controls plasma uridine levels.

However, the system goes offline when you start fasting. The liver changes personality and becomes primarily concerned with keeping blood sugar levels up. Sorry, shop's closed, no uridine for sale. Fat cells pick up the slack and start begging for food by pumping uridine in the bloodstream directly. The uridine pours into the brain from fat cells and signals the hypothalamus to turn down your internal thermostat and go into shutdown mode.[9] This results in a small drop in body temperature like what happens in hibernating mammals. This protective response probably exists to slow metabolism and ease

NAD+ demands. It could also provide some protection from increasing oxidation in the mitochondria. Fat cells that are busy producing uridine during fasting have to stop making leptin, a hunger-controlling hormone that also works in the hypothalamus. This may be why people have trouble with hunger and weight gain after gall bladder removal. Uridine just streams into the circulation directly like water from a leaking dike. This may also be why fasting is so difficult to pull off. Mmmmm . . . doughnuts.

## THE HUNGER GAINS

Okay, so you've heard enough and you want to try a little fasting. That's cool, but you'll need to pick which *kind* of fasting. One way is to sharply cut your daily caloric intake (by 10 to 40 percent) like McCay's rats. You could also intermittently fast. In 1945, a University of Chicago study found that fasting on alternate days improved the health of their test animals and lengthened their lives. This was revisited by the University of Illinois at Chicago in a 2017 study where researchers compared alternate-day fasting with daily calorie restriction.[10] What happened? Not a whole lot. No difference was seen between the two groups. Both had improved health indicators and similar, modest weight loss (about 6 percent). More people dropped out of the fasting group.

Another variation of the alternating routine is to slash calories to 25 percent of the normal intake 1 day but then get to scarf up 125 percent the next day. When folks on this feast-or-famine regimen were compared in a 1-year study to those who cut their daily diet by 25 percent, no differences were seen. Both groups were healthier and lost a little weight (6 percent). Oh, there was one difference. The fasting group had way more dropouts. That whole hunger thing.

One popular form of intermittent fasting is to sprinkle 2 days during the week when you consume only 500 to 600 calories, a 5-2 deal. Another new alternative is a "CR-mimetic" or "fasting-mimetic diet" that allows people to eat a normal diet for most of the month, but then limits them for 5 days a month to a 700- to 1,100-calorie restricted diet high in unsaturated fats, low in carbohydrates, and low in proteins. Mice did well on this diet, living longer and getting fewer tumors. In a 3-month human trial of the diet published in early 2017, UCLA biochemist Valter Longo noted an average 6-pound weight loss, lower blood sugar, and lower total cholesterol.[11] Not unexpectedly, insulin-like growth factor-1 (IGF-1) serum levels increased in the test subjects, reflecting metabolic stress in the liver. The good thing is that IGF-1 binding protein production went up even higher, effectively lowering serum IGF-1 levels, theoretically protecting cellular integrity and sentinel disease monitoring.

Because your internal circadian clock is connected to metabolism, the timing of your meals is important. In fact, the easiest entryway to fasting is to just tighten up your meal times. Rather than grazing all day, eat only during a limited period. Time-restricted feeding (TRF) has been shown to help control weight gain and improve health indices in animal and early human pilot studies.[12] Researchers have also found that mice who were fed a high-fat diet with time restrictions remained thinner and healthier than control mice who grazed all day. The first human trials of time-restricted feeding have been promising. A 2017 Italian study found that combining resistance training with TRF (without calorie restriction) for an 8-hour period was particularly beneficial with decreased blood lipids, glucose, insulin, and inflammation, as well as rapid weight loss without loss of strength.[13] The researchers found an increase in blood adiponectin in the TRF group, a possible reason for the improvement in metabolic indicators. Adiponectin triggers AMPK activity and peroxisome proliferator-activated receptor-gamma coactivator 1-alpha (PGC-1alpha), which cause jumps in mitochondrial biogenesis and energy expenditure in the brain and muscular tissue.[14]

The best way to try this kind of fasting is to hold off eating for 4 hours after waking up *and* 4 hours before you sleep. Call it the 4-hour rule (Figure 5). The process leverages your circadian rhythm and sleep cycle to ease the pain, leaving most adults with a functional 8- to 10-hour window to work with. This can work even without cutting calories, but works way better if you push back a little. Oh, and no grazing allowed. Too harsh for you? Consider it more of a guideline than a rule. Pick one 4-hour block—morning or night—and at least restrict your meals to the remaining 12 hours. Work the night shift? No problem, just adjust the bezel on the clock, and the

4-hour rule can still help you improve metabolism and control hunger.

The most surprising thing about fasting compared to other diets is that it doesn't result in substantial long-term weight loss. There might be some early decrease in weight, but the body's metabolism is ruthlessly stable, and energy balance rules the day. If you stop fasting, any weight loss you gained will slowly be lost. Still, fasting does offer some definite benefits. You can expect les inflammation, better glucose tolerance, lower blood pressure, and maybe even a longer life.[15] There are many ways you can unlock the benefits of fasting. Try cutting your calories in half 1 day a week or maybe give time-restricted feeding a go, like I do. Whatever type of fasting you do choose, it has a much better chance of working if it feels natural and easy to you.

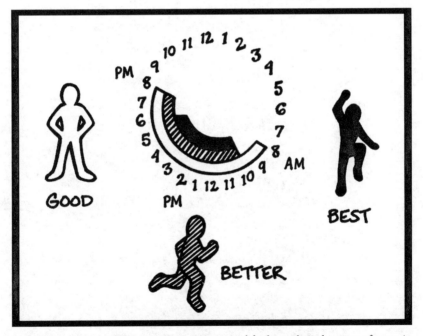

**FIGURE 5: THE 4-HOUR RULE.** Time-restricted feeding takes advantage of your circadian rhythms to give you the benefits of fasting and calorie restriction without all the sacrifice and hunger pains. Try to limit all your meals to a 12-hour or less stretch for optimal metabolic efficiency and health benefits. Twist the bezel of this dial to fit your work schedule if you pull the night shift. (*Illustration: Jacob Scheyder*)

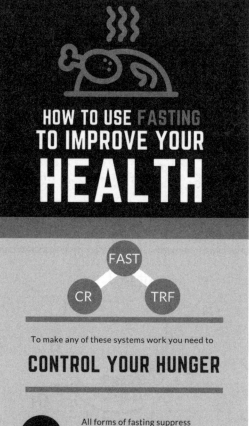

## HOW TO USE FASTING TO IMPROVE YOUR HEALTH

FAST

CR          TRF

To make any of these systems work you need to

## CONTROL YOUR HUNGER

**FAST** — All forms of fasting suppress mTORC and ramp up metabolism. The simplest way is to just skip eating once a week.

**CR** — Calorie restriction doesn't just mean skipping a meal here or there. You need to slash daily caloric intake to less than 1,800 per day.

**TRF** — Time-restricted feeding leverages circadian rhythms to get the benefits of fasting. Get all your meals knocked out in 8 to 12 hours and you don't have to cut calories.

VERDICT? TRF IS THE BEST.

# 5

# HACKING THE GENOME

"Big things have small beginnings."

—T. E. LAWRENCE, *LAWRENCE OF ARABIA*, 1962

**SOME OF MAN'S GREATEST** technical achievements were born in war. It is fitting, then, that the greatest scientific breakthrough of this young century would be the result of the most ancient of struggles—the battle between bacteria and viruses. The discovery of CRISPR gene editing techniques offers the ability to selectively remove defective genes and replace them with corrected versions. This could allow precise genetic surgery before organ failure sets in. Some of the most devastating genetic illnesses, such as Duchenne muscular dystrophy, Tay-Sachs disease, and Huntington's disease, could be treated with targeted genetic editing. The theoretical implications are clear: a longer, healthier life. The problem is that gene editing is truly Pandora's box. It could enhance an athlete's performance, a scientist's analytic processing, or a soldier's strength. Splicing genes into germinal cells like sperm and eggs is even more provocative, since it could conceivably lead to directed, accelerated human evolution. Hold on, people. Before you start stressing out about designer babies and super soldiers, let's take a quick look at the history of the CRISPR craze.

## PASSPORT, PLEASE

In 1987, Yoshizumi Ishino and his group at Osaka University made a strange discovery while studying the genes of E. coli bacteria.[1] They found long repetitive sequence buried in the DNA of single-celled bacteria. As metagenomics developed over the next 2 decades, gene sequencing became increasingly sophisticated, and many more of these strange stretches of DNA were discovered. In 2002, Dutch scientist Ruud Jansen named them CRISPR, short for clustered regularly interspaced short palindromic repeats. He and his colleagues at Utrecht University also noticed that they were always located near to genes that coded for DNA-cutting enzymes, dubbed *cas* proteins. In 2005, CRISPR DNA sequences were discovered in bacteria that exactly matched the DNA codes of viruses they battled with.[2] This confirmed what scientists had suspected: Bacteria have their own adaptive immune system.

It has been long known that bacteria have restriction enzymes that are triggered to blow up when exposed to DNA unprotected by a nucleus. This innate immunity usually occurs when a virus attaches to the bacterial wall and injects the bacteria with a dose of naked viral DNA or plasmid. Adaptive immunity kicks in when an infected microbe survives with a copy of the viral DNA locked in its genome. The next time the microbe is attacked by the same virus, it reads the DNA barcode and the cas enzyme chops it up to prevent viral replication. This is analogous to our human adaptive immune response that occurs when our white cells eat invaders and spit out bits of proteins called antigens. These antigens then generate antibodies that allow us to adapt to future attacks. Since these changes do not occur in germinal cells, we can't pass our adaptive immunity to our children. Bacteria can.

When they divide, microbes pass down this

> **WHERE DID CRISPR COME FROM?**
> CRISPR evolved as a primitive immune system in bacteria buried in their DNA that they use to identify and kill viruses that have attacked their ancestors in the past. Scientists use CRISPR today to splice genes in any organism they want. What could go wrong?

viral DNA copy. This hacked genetic memory increases over time as the bacterial colonies are exposed to more viral infections. Genetic analyses of common bacteria have detected thousands of DNA signatures of current and extinct viruses in a multimillion-year-old evolutionary defense tree. CRISPR-mediated immunity may be only the beginning. A new theory suggests that microbes use CRISPR not only to identify viral invaders, but also to identify each other. Bacteria have DNA runs called mobile elements that allow them to copy their own DNA and infect a host directly or remotely by sticking their DNA into a drone virus. Eugene V. Koonin and Mart Krupovic of the Pasteur Institute found a group of mobile elements called casposons that may be the forerunners of DNA-cutting cas enzymes.[3] In this way, CRISPR DNA runs might act as cellular passports. Microbes could also use CRISPR sequences to identify each other or to silence some of their own genes—like making fake IDs to hide and survive in hostile environments.

## PLAYING WITH FIRE

No matter what the true nature of CRISPR is in the wild, its domestication is driving a revolution. The power of this simple technique to transform our lives is unprecedented. The dairy industry has always been dependent on healthy bacterial colonies to make cheese and yogurt. The problem has been that viral infections could cause expensive losses of bacterial lines. After the discovery of CRISPR-cas, Rodolphe Barrangou, a microbiologist working for Danisco, creatively used this adaptive immunity to tackle the problem.[4] He took milk and mixed it with streptococcus infected with no viral strains. While the viruses killed many of the bacteria, the ones that survived incorporated slugs of viral DNA and became resistant to them. If the researchers cut out the CRISPR viral DNA copies, the bacteria lost their immunity. Now most dairy manufacturers use CRISPR-mediated adaptive immunity to protect their yogurt and cheese production. The FDA doesn't consider gene editing to be the same as transgenic insertion, so no GMO label for you.

In 2012, Jennifer Doudna, Emmanuelle Charpantier, and their colleagues took this CRISPR tech to another level.[5] They attached a guiding piece of RNA to a CRISPR-cas9 complex and used it like a guided missile to enter a microbe and precisely cut its DNA at the spot that matched the guide RNA (Figure 6). The CRISPR-cas9 complex could be used as a tool to regulate and edit genes like a molecular Pacman. This breakthrough spawned hundreds of gene splicing experiments around the world using CRISPR-cas9 to target, cut, and replace DNA sequences. Scientists have now used CRISPR-cas9 probes to successfully treat HIV, hepatitis B, and age-related macular degeneration.

CRISPR-cas9 technology allows labs to create genetically edited "knockout" mice with dramatic speed compared to the expensive, traditional process of homologous recombination. Knockout mice are critical in the biomedical world because they allow researchers to test the effects of gene deletion or modification directly. Traditionally, this is a long, tedious process called homologous recombination. Using this technique, a mouse

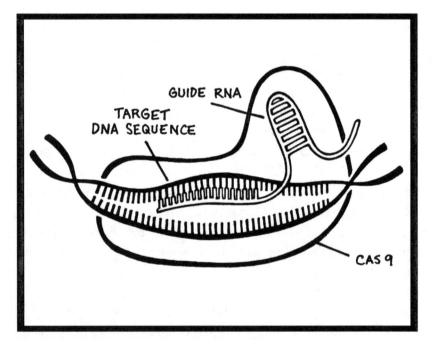

**FIGURE 6: GENE SPLICING 101.** CRISPR-cas9 hunts the target DNA sequence, unzips the ladder, and inserts the new command code. After CRISPR undocks and bails out, the natural host repair mechanisms take over, and the altered gene is integrated. (*Illustration: Jacob Scheyder*)

embryo would be seeded with the altered DNA, and the first generation produced would be chimera who had a mixture of normal and altered DNA. If a chimera with the altered DNA in their sperm mated, eventually you would get one with altered DNA. Then you would have to successfully breed a pair of mixed DNA mice together, etc., until you got your mutant mouse ready. This process takes more than a year and tens of thousands of dollars. CRISPR-cas9 radically changed this process since you could inject it directly into the embryo. This could edit all the genes at once and produce a knock-out mouse in one generation.

CRISPR-cas9 is also way more effective than other commonly used gene editors, transcription activator-like effector nucleases (TALENs) and zinc finger nuclease (ZFN). Although they recognize longer DNA sequences than CRISPR-cas9, they require constant customization and experimentation to get the right recombinant result. CRISPR is so good at editing that you can use it to insert any type of information into DNA for storage. George Church's group at Harvard was even able to use CRISPR to insert a movie clip into bacterial DNA and retrieve it intact.[6] A movie!

As good as CRISPR-cas9 has been as a gene editor, it is only just beginning to realize its full potential as a gene reader. New techniques have allowed scientists to hack the hacker. By essentially breaking the cas9 cutting enzyme, researchers can use the CRISPR-cas9 complex to locate and attach itself to any gene they want. By attaching an activator protein to the dead cas9 enzyme, they can turn the gene on or off. They can even stick it to a fluorescent marker to make it glow when activated. The ability to stack the system with different commands has allowed researchers around the world to explore the epigenetic control of the genome by turning multiple genes on and off in various combinations, opening the way to meaningful gene therapy.

## A BETTER MOUSETRAP

Age-related macular degeneration (AMD) is one of the most common causes of blindness, affecting 10 percent of people over age 65. The primary cause of AMD is overproduction of vascular endothelial growth factor (VEGF). This creates a rat nest of vascular clumps that leak and bleed, blocking the central macular portion of the retina. A team from the Seoul Center for Genome Engineering has used CRISPR-cas9 injections directly into the diseased retinal epithelium to cut out the VEGF gene, which quickly begins to clear the retinal damage.[7] Great, right? Like a genetic scalpel. Not quite. New work from Columbia University on reversing blindness in mice using CRISPR-cas9 revealed that the system is not as precise as previously thought.[8] When correcting a mutation in the Pde6b gene, CRISPR-cas9 editing caused more than 1,500 unintended genetic mutations and 100 unexpected gene deletions/additions. With human trials of CRISPR-cas9 under way in China and more planned in the United States, this has created alarm. These concerns as well as ongoing legal struggles over who owns the patent rights to CRISPR-cas9 have helped fuel the demand for competing, more precise DNA gene-splicing systems.

These include a smaller but more efficient DNA-snipping enzyme called Cpf1 discovered in common bacteria. This has already been used by scientists from the University of Texas in cultured human heart cells to correct mutant genes that cause Duchenne muscular dystrophy, a devastating degenerative muscle disease.[9] CRISPR-Cpf1 has several advantages over cas9. It is smaller since it does not require a second strand of extra tracer RNA, and can enter the cell more easily. It also makes a staggered DNA cut, making it more precise than the blunt-cutting cas9 enzyme. Because Cpf1 cuts the DNA away from the edited gene, the "seed" region is safer and more effectively preserved. In China, where work on nonviable human embryos has started, a new system similar to CRISPR, called NgAgo, has been used. Many more gene-editing CRISPR-cas variants are on the way as the technology expands into crop and livestock management.

## DARK MATTERS

Remember all that junk DNA we talked about? If only about 2 percent of our DNA codes for proteins, what does the more than 98 percent do? CRISPR-cas gene readers may help solve this mystery. We know that all this genetic "dark matter" must have some purpose. Some of this DNA may represent extended sequences of noncoding RNA and microRNA that could function to modify the risk of common diseases or epigenetic gene regulation. By using CRISPR to modify long stretches of regulatory DNA, researchers are beginning to map this uncharted genetic country.

The real work of CRISPR systems has just started as it converges with stem cell research.[10] Stem cells are primitive, pluripotent cells that can grow up to be any of a different line of adult cells, such as skin, bone, cartilage, muscle, etc. Stem cells were first manipulated in 1962 in an experiment that created shock and disbelief at the time. John Gurdon at Cambridge University took the cellular nucleus of an adult frog and injected it into a frog egg without a nucleus. The egg reset the epigenetic clock of the adult nucleus, driving it back into an embryonic state. This chimera then went on to develop into an otherwise normal-appearing tadpole. This led to the gradual adoption of cloning technology, culminating in the birth of Dolly the sheep in 1992. The ethical whiplash this created was widespread, leading to extensive cloning and stem cell growth restrictions in the United States adopted during the Bush years that are still in place. Despite the early success of cloning and creating pluripotent stem cell lines, many mysteries remain. Manipulation of stem cells has traditionally been difficult, requiring the use of retroviruses used to insert the DNA code changes. Now that CRISPR has arrived, the two technologies have begun to blend synergistically.

Chronic granulomatous disease is a serious genetic disorder with few treatment options. It usually leads to the need for long-term antibiotics and long-term risk of lethal infection due to a defect in the NOX2 protein. Previous attempts at stem cell treatment have been risky and even deadly. Suk See De Ravin of the National Institutes of Health and colleagues used CRISPR-cas9 gene editing to successfully repair hematopoietic stem cells from patients with X-linked chronic granulomatous disease and transplant them to mice, where they survived and functioned well without side effects.[11]

## GODS AND KINGS

What signals were triggered in Gurdon's tadpole eggs to allow the cytoplasm to reset the nuclear DNA motherboard, essentially turning an adult into a fetus? The mystery remained unsolved for almost 5 decades. In 2006, Shinya Yamanaka and his colleagues at Japan's Kyoto University discovered four transcriptional genes in the dark void of DNA that could trigger the journey back to the embryonic state.[12] These four genes, Oct14, Sox2, Kif4, and c-Myc, now called Yamanaka factors, are considered master genes that can turn any adult cell into an induced pluripotent stem cell (ipSC).

Their revolutionary work led to Yamanaka and Gurdon being awarded the Nobel Prize in 2012. When later researchers tried giving Yamanaka factor cocktails to adult mice, however, they met with disaster. The mice developed tumors or metabolic diseases and died. A group at the Salk Institute led by Juan Carlos Izpisua Belmonte kept working. By cutting back the Yamanaka gene factor dosage given to age-accelerated mice ravaged by progeria, they finally succeeded.[13] The mice not only survived, but they lived 30 percent longer and showed invigorated health. More importantly, the researchers found improved metabolic health in a group of normal middle-aged rodents fed the same power shake. Their epigenetic programs were being at least partially over-written without sending them on a Benjamin Button trip back to a primordial pile of goo. Aging could be reversed.

Despite all the obstacles, the main brake on all this research has been those pesky ethical issues. A science advisory group from the National Academy of Sciences and the National Academy of Medicine released a statement on human gene editing supporting work if prohibitions were placed to prevent alterations resembling "enhancement" and other "off-label" applications. The only problem is that it never specified who would police all this fun.[14] Eventually, we will be able to modify stem cells to do whatever we want. Don't think so? Congenital cardiomyopathy is a cruel disease. It's an autosomal dominant

## CAN STEM CELL TREATMENTS CURE ARTHRITIS?

Adults have a small number of stem cells in every tissue. Federal law prevents the culturing of harvested adult stem cells to crank that number up. This limits the possibility of stem cell success. Once you develop a bowleg (varus) or knock-knee (valgus) knee alignment, your knee is shot and it's time for some titanium and plastic. So, the answer is no.

mutation, meaning that it takes just one copy gene to screw you over and destroy your heart. Just one. Hypertrophic cardiomyopathy is a degenerative disease that affects 1 out of every 500 adults and is a leading cause of sudden cardiac death in young athletes. The muscle spindles are defective, leading to left ventricular hypertrophy and cardiac muscle disarray. Basically, your heart strangles itself. The terrible thing is that this type of mutation is a silent one that selectively involves myosin binding protein C-cardiac (MYBPC3); you don't even know that you have it until after you've passed it down to your kids. Genetics can suck. The autosomal dominant breast cancer mutations BRCA1 and BRCA2 are another pair of sneaky bastards like MYBPC3. An international group of genetic engineers used a slick experimental model with CRISPR-cas9 to edit and correct the MYBPC3 genetic mutation and cure idiopathic cardiomyopathy in viable embryos with a 73 percent success rate.[15]

That's damn awesome, but where do we draw the thin CRISPR line? Once you start messing with germinal cell lines like sperm cells and eggs, you start to change the species. That's some pretty sketchy stuff. Even if we just stick to your basic adult stem cells, the ethical questions are legion. Stem cell exhaustion (particularly in the hypothalamus) is one of the hallmarks of aging. It is conceivable that with modified stem cell edit-shots targeting the hypothalamus you could extend human health and life— indefinitely. At least for those who could afford it. After watching my wife balancing our last bank statement, I'm guessing I won't be one of them.

Or maybe I will. The coolest, all-time scariest aspect of this DNA coding frenzy is its democracy. Anybody can edit genes. Anybody. Got a little dough and some extra space in your dusty old garage? Go for it. The gene-splicing industry is completely unregulated. You can hop online and pick up a starter CRISPR-cas9 DIY kit for under 99 bucks. Canadian. Okay, maybe it's not that cheap or easy. At least for now you are not going to be able to whip up a *Yamankale* shake to score yourself some more good years. A little genetic nip and tuck isn't waiting on tonight's dance card. Luckily, now that you understand the power of metabolism, we can start hacking our DNA the old-fashioned way by eating right and hitting the gym. With a hormone chaser.

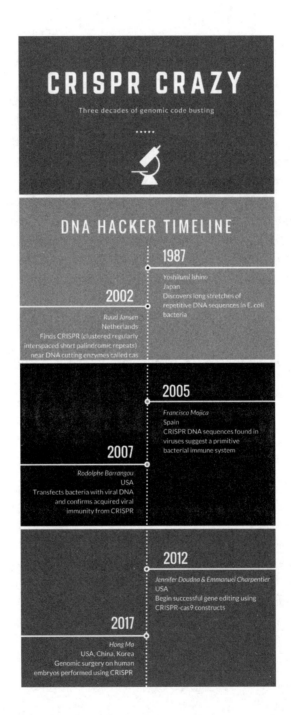

# CRISPR CRAZY

Three decades of genomic code busting

• • • • •

## DNA HACKER TIMELINE

### 1987
*Yoshilumi Ishino*
Japan
Discovers long stretches of
repetitive DNA sequences in E. coli
bacteria

### 2002
*Ruud Jansen*
Netherlands
Finds CRISPR (clustered regularly
interspaced short palindromic repeats)
near DNA cutting enzymes called cas

### 2005
*Francisco Mojica*
Spain
CRISPR DNA sequences found in
viruses suggest a primitive
bacterial immune system

### 2007
*Rodolphe Barrangou*
USA
Transfects bacteria with viral DNA
and confirms acquired viral
immunity from CRISPR

### 2012
*Jennifer Doudna & Emmanuel Charpentier*
USA
Begin successful gene editing using
CRISPR-cas9 constructs

### 2017
*Hong Ma*
USA, China, Korea
Genomic surgery on human
embryos performed using CRISPR

# PHASE TWO
## DIET

# 6

# BRIDGE OF LIES

"In science, error always precedes the truth, and it is better it should go first rather than last."

—HUGH WALPOLE, *THE WOODEN HORSE*, 1909

**WE LIVE IN STRANGE** times. Man is at war with food. As in most conflicts, we have vilified our enemies—cholesterol, fat, sugar, salt, and even wheat. We have spent extraordinary amounts of time, money, and sacrifice over the past century to control our environment and throttle our appetites. Despite substantial expenditures, we are losing. Sixty years after the American Medical Association declared obesity a national crisis, we are heavier than ever. Today, 155 million Americans are overweight, and obesity causes more deaths every year than smoking.[1] The answer must be simple. Eat less and exercise more, right? Wrong. The mantra of the past 6 decades has failed. The answers to this riddle are complex, but we are now armed with new research on nutrition and fitness that can finally help. More importantly, we have started questioning the dietary dogma that we used to blindly accept.

In the first section of *The Fountain,* we gained fresh perspectives about how the body's metabolism works. Humans are driven by energy and error. Our bodies strive for efficiency and labor to maintain balance. In the end, food is not our enemy. Calories do not have personalities. Macronutrients are not evil. Myths and oversimplifications are what have driven us to where we are. For the longest time we've been at war with ourselves, and it is finally time for a ceasefire. To have fit and healthy bodies, we must start using our biggest evolutionary advantage—our brains.

## BON SAUVAGE

There is a general belief that obesity and its resultant health risks, including type 2 diabetes, cancer, and heart disease, are the result of the spread of a sedentary Western lifestyle marked by inactivity and dietary excess. Many people believe that it is this divergence from our evolutionary roots as foraging Paleolithic hunter-gatherers that has been our undoing. Cars and cellphones replaced spears and sickles. Surely, a sturdy African bushman hunting down game must burn more calories than a fluffy Wall Street hedge fund manager. The problem is that this simply isn't true. Anthropologist Herman Pontzer and his colleagues at Hunter College traveled to Tanzania to study the metabolic rate and energy consumption of the primitive Hadza, one of the world's few remaining hunter-gatherer tribes, and compare them to their Western contemporaries.[2] Their findings were striking. Despite dramatic lifestyle differences, pound for pound, there was little or no difference between the Hadza and a broad range of cultures in how many calories they burned daily.

This makes sense when viewed through the prism of metabolism. Man evolved in calorie-restricted environments where high levels of physical activity were needed to find food. This forced our bodies to evolve sophisticated thermostatic control of our metabolism. When muscular demands increase, energy use in other parts of the bodies must diminish to maintain balance. Metabolism *decreases* to reset the caloric thermostat. When you combine severe calorie restriction with exercise, your metabolism slows down even more to conserve energy levels. Nutritional researcher Kevin

Hall and his colleagues at the National Institutes of Health tracked metabolic adaptations of contestants from the reality show *The Biggest Loser*.[3] Even though the contestants averaged an initial weight loss of 127 pounds each and kept up an exercise program, their metabolism gradually adapted by slowing way down and never increased. They gained back most of the lost weight over the following 6 years.

This is the main reason exercise alone is not an effective way to lose weight. You might trick the system into burning some readily available fat stores for a few weeks, but your muscles and metabolism quickly recalibrate and become more efficient to reset the caloric thermostat.[4] The message is clear: We have evolved to have a relatively stable metabolic rate that resists change. The interesting thing is that the number one consumer of energy in our body is our brain. It sucks up 80 percent of our caloric resources. The whole evolutionary point of all this metabolic balance is to preserve the energy pipeline to this most important organ. Okay, maybe the second most important one.

How do you work with your inner tribesman? Look, you just can't outrun a cupcake. The USDA estimates that we consume 25 percent more calories than we did in 1970. That certainly doesn't help. Metabolism respects the first law of thermodynamics, and energy must be conserved. However, our systems are thermodynamically open and aren't perfectly efficient. A body that is unhealthy is going to waste even more precious energetic resources repairing mounting metabolic errors. Working out is critical to staying healthy, and we do know muscle uses more energy than fat—one reason strength training helps burn serious calories. But working out by itself is not going to make you much thinner. You have to control the amount of fuel you are piping into your beautiful machine. Respect the base energy needs of the body and understand that weight loss through caloric restriction is a painfully slow process, but it can be done. The good news is that you'll have to knock off only about 5 percent of your weight to gain most of the health benefits of weight loss.

We are metabolically flexible. It's how humans can survive and even thrive in extreme environments. Although the popular Paleolithic diet, high in proteins and stripped of dairy, grains, and potatoes, might be better than loading up on fast food, it's a fake. We evolved to eat what is available. In a brilliant commentary on the subject, paleoanthropologist Peter Ungar correctly pointed out how geography has driven the dramatically different diets of the isolated Tikigagmiut tribe of northern Alaska, who eat a sea-based diet of protein and saturated fat, and the Gwi San of southern Africa, who instead get most of their calories from a diet rich in carbohydrates from roots and fruits.[5] Yet, both groups have survived. How can this work? Our true evolutionary gift may not be in our brains, but in our genes. Our basic genetic code is triggered to change and adapt by our environment and diet to help us maintain metabolic balance. We have many ways to distill nutrients and make the energy we need to survive. Even our gut flora changes its population mix to adapt. The trick is to learn from our ancestors—not to mimic them. Then we can pick our battles and make good, healthy choices when it comes to food. For example, there are aspects of our diet that are far less important than we have been taught. Like fat.

## BIG FAT LIARS

Let's chew the fat a little. When we have more calories than we need, we convert them into fat. The human body uses this stored fat to stockpile energy. When we need a power-up, we can readily access it and burn it off to make ATP. Fat cells also make leptin, a hormone that streams into the brain to control hunger. But there are other kinds of fatty acids that we cannot make and need to consume. The essential fatty acids, specifically omega-6 fatty acid (linoleic acid) and omega-3 fatty acid (alpha-linolenic acid), were discovered in 1923. We need these guys to make cellular membranes and insulate our porous electrical systems. Our nerves are coated in fatty acid–based myelin sheaths, and our brains are nearly 60 percent fat. We also use essential fatty acids to metabolize cholesterol, make hormones, keep our blood pressure in check, and basically grease the wheels. Men need 17 grams of omega-3 and 1.6 grams of omega-6 a day, while women need 11 grams and 1.1 grams in their daily diet.

In general, there are four types of fat: saturated fats, unsaturated fats, monosaturated fats, and trans fats. All dietary fat contains a *blend* of these different fatty acids. For example, corn oil is considered a polyunsaturated fat but contains a mix of 24 percent monosaturated fatty acids and 59 percent polyunsaturated fatty acids. Fatty acids are basically long chains of linked carbons that vary in length but invariably end in a carboxyl (COOH) group. The amount of saturation refers to the number of hydrogen atoms stuck to the long carbon chains. Increasing hydrogen saturation thickens up the fatty acids by raising their melting point. Saturated fats are found in meat, fish, egg yolks, chocolate, and tropical oils. Unsaturated fats are like those in vegetable oils. Monosaturated fats are more prevalent in olive oil.

Both saturated and unsaturated fats are naturally produced, but trans fats were created in a laboratory where plant oils and metal were heated together to extreme temperatures in a vacuum. The process was discovered by Paul Sabatier when he was able to partially hydrogenate oil vapors in the 1890s. In 1901, German chemist Wilhelm Normann modified the technique to partially hydrogenate liquid oils while trying to make soap. The result was too greasy to be used as soap, but boy did it make damn fine fried chicken. In 1911, Proctor & Gamble bought the US patent rights to Normann's process and introduced the world to Crisco—short for *crystallized cotton seed oil*. In 1912, Paul Sabatier was awarded the Nobel Prize in biochemistry for the discovery of trans fats. Thanks, man.

> **DOES SATURATED FAT CAUSE HEART DISEASE?**
>
> No. Heart disease results from senescent cells that burrow into the walls of arteries and induce inflammation. Gentlemen, remember that you need dietary cholesterol to make testosterone.

For the past 70 years, we have been told that saturated fats, the kind found in meat and dairy products along with cholesterol, are lethal. The link between diet and heart disease was first raised in a study by Ancel Keys at the University of Minnesota in 1947 and later was expanded to the widely influential, but flawed, Seven Countries Study in 1957.[6, 7] The diet-heart hypothesis reasons that saturated animal fat leads to high levels of cholesterol in the blood, which deposit in the coronary arteries to form plaques that choke off bloodflow in the heart or chip off and clog brain arteries, leading to potentially catastrophic strokes. By the end of the decade, the American Heart Association and USDA joined forces to identify saturated fats as public enemy number one—the primary cause of heart disease, high blood pressure, strokes, and death—and pushed hard to decrease their use.

So, what did our national health advocates do? They gave us substitutes. Based on little data and research funded by industrial advocacy groups, like the Wesson (Oil) Fund for Medical Research, the door opened to a dramatic increase in the use of polyunsaturated oil and even cheaper industrial trans fats in processed foods like margarine and fast food. The theory was simple—simply slide vegetable oils high in linoleic acid (like corn oil) into the American diet, and serum cholesterol would drop. With cholesterol finally mastered, the risk of heart disease and death from cardiovascular disease would evaporate. Most of the data to support this diet-heart hypothesis was observational, pooled from years of participant questionnaires, interviews, and surveys. You know, the reliable kind of data you'd be willing to risk your life on. Even as the highly publicized Senate subcommittee meetings on nutrition and heart disease wrapped up in 1977 with a new FDA fiat endorsing a low-fat/high complex carbohydrate national diet, serious doubts were already being raised.[8]

It was in this controversial context that the Minnesota Coronary Survey led by Irving Frantz, a physiologist from the University of Minnesota and early proponent of the saturated fat-cholesterol-heart attack-death cycle, was reaching completion. The study was a massive undertaking to measure the effects of replacing saturated fat with unsaturated fat that was funded by the National Institutes of Health (NIH) from 1968 to 1973. A rarity in nutritional research even by today's standards, the study was prospective, double-blind, and randomized. Granted, it's old data, but Level I evidence in 1977 is still Level 1 evidence in 2017. The subjects were all either residents of the Oak Terrace retirement home or shuttered in one of six state-run mental institutions. The groups were divided equally into men and women ages 20 to 97 and were further divided equally into control and test groups *without informed consent.* Just wait, the ethical freefall of this study is just beginning. The control group ate a standard diet of the time with 18 percent saturated fat while the test group ate a diet with 10 percent of these saturated fats replaced by polyunsaturated fat (corn oil) and half the cholesterol content. All the authors had to do was wait for the control group to start dropping like flies after a few years of the high-test diet and their hypothesis would be proven. But that's not what happened.

In 1989, a full 16 years after the study's conclusion, a terse six-page report was finally released in which the authors reported a 14 percent decrease in cholesterol levels in the test group and concluded that "no differences between the treatment and control groups were observed for cardiovascular events, cardiovascular deaths, or total mortality."[9] In 2009, Frantz died and his secrets might have been lost forever. In 2013, Christopher Ramsden, an NIH researcher with a gift for forensic data reconstruction, contacted Frantz's sons, both physicians, who helped recover boxes of dusty old IBM tapes that contained the carefully documented records and original data from the study's 9,423 participants.[10] They corroborated the initial claims of a 14 percent decline in serum cholesterol levels. However, as the subjects' cholesterol levels dropped, their risk of dying *increased.* For every 30-point decline in cholesterol, the death risk increased by 22 percent—a fact suppressed in the original report. Now that's some serious data flexibility. How could lowering cholesterol with polyunsaturated fats increase your chances of dying? Long chain fatty acids are metabolized into smaller acids that can cause inflammatory and oxidative damage to the heart and other tissue.[11]

Ramsden and his team also performed a meta-analysis of all the available randomized controlled studies where saturated fats were substituted with polyunsaturated fats, and they reached the same conclusions.[12] Cholesterol levels dropped, but deaths from heart disease and stroke remained about the same. In 2015, another landmark review of pooled prospective studies from Russell de Souza and his team at Canada's McMaster University found similar results.[13] Although they did find a possible causal relationship with trans fats, saturated fats were not associated with any increase in mortality, cardiovascular disease, stroke, type 2 diabetes, or stroke rates. While many studies have shown that replacing saturated fat with linoleic acid (vegetable oil) lowers serum cholesterol levels, no study has ever presented direct evidence that this lowers the risk of heart attacks or death from heart disease.[14]

Why? Atherosclerosis and heart disease are *inflammatory* disorders.[15] Cholesterol plaques form, macrophages come in to chew them up, they eat their fill, form giant fat-laden foam cells, and they die . . . creating more inflammation. It's like a giant zit forming in your left main coronary artery ready to pop at any moment. Yikes. What do we do? There is no real clinical evidence to prove that saturated fat is either good or bad for you. Your go-to hangover-busting omelet is still in the game. Substituting carbohydrates for saturated fats only worsens the problem, since it can lead to insulin resistance and obesity—two prime suspects that might worsen inflammatory vascular damage.

As for industrial trans fats, don't worry, our nimble-footed FDA decided to ban them in 2015. But the ban doesn't start until 2018. Apparently, the food industry needed 3 years to come up with an alternate way to make Twinkies. Just after the ban was approved, a study was published in the *European Heart Journal* showing that natural trans fats and low levels of industrial trans fats had no impact on cardiovascular disease rates in Germany.[16]

If you're like me and have high cholesterol no matter what you eat, the problem is even more complicated. We just don't have the cellular biotech to process it (thanks, Pops). Luckily for us, a statin pill can solve what the most stringent diets can't—correct our lousy LDL to HDL ratio and slow down plaque formation. As for those senescent foam cells already lurking in the creases of our coronaries, senolytic medications are just around the corner to flush the system. Today, many cardiologists now advise a Mediterranean diet emphasizing unprocessed food laced with plant-based saturated fats combined with 30 minutes a day of intense exercise to keep your pipes clean. Will this work for everyone? Probably not. As with all dietary studies, a grain of salt is needed. In 2013, a highly publicized trial of a Mediterranean-style diet projected a 30 percent decrease in cardiovascular deaths.[17] However, as researcher Jerome Groopman pointed out in 2017, this was a little statistical skullduggery since the Med diet subjects traded their olive oil and nuts for less than a 1 percent survival advantage over the control group.[18] Though this finding doesn't mean you should skip your workout and start adding a side of Crisco to your steak and potato dinner.

There is one more reason men need to keep some fat in our diet. Hormones, gentlemen. Testosterone and cortisol are needed for healthy muscle metabolism. When you strip a diet of fatty acids, testosterone and cortisol levels plummet. A study that compared a 20 percent fat diet (polyunsaturated fat in oils) with a 40 percent fat diet (animal sourced) found much lower testosterone levels in the 20 percent fat subjects.[19] When the researchers switched the lower-fat intake subjects up to a 40 percent fat diet, their testosterone levels rapidly recovered. Hormones are very sensitive to dietary and training stress. Testosterone and adrenal cortisol production plummet with low-carbohydrate diets, high-protein diets, vegan diets, and even endurance training.[20] High-intensity resistance exercise seems to at least partially protect your testosterone and cortisol reservoirs from the siphoning effects of radical dieting.

## SWEET REVENGE

Our relationship with sugar has always been conflicted. After all, we metabolize all the food we consume to a sugar, glucose, to produce all the energy needed for life. Ribose, another sugar, forms the backbone of our protein-making RNA strands. Even the most basic of all sugars, glucaldehyde, an ancient building block of ribose, is found throughout the Milky Way. We need sugars. But man evolved in a world where food resources were scarce, so it's no wonder we learned to crave sweet things. To feed our growing, gas-guzzling brains, we developed a finely tuned sweet tooth and metabolic flexibility to survive. Our neurons dig sugar, rewarding us with a dose of dopamine in exchange to encourage the hunt. Even primitive hunter-gatherer tribes like the Hadza of Tanzania and the Mbuti of the Congo still shift to diets based predominately on honey and fruit sugar during their long rainy seasons.

Our obsession with sugar is hardwired into our brains and has shaped our civilization from the beginning. Neolithic man's first crops were sweet; figs and sugarcane were domesticated more than 11,000 years ago. Later, sugar from condensed Arabian honey was used as a medicine in ancient Rome. The first sugar crystals were produced in India around 350 AD, and sugar refining spread throughout the Near and Far East. Crusaders brought sugarcane with them back to Europe to supplement honey as a sweetener.[21] Labor-intense sugar mills proliferated in the 1400s and contributed to the growth of the African slave trade in Spain and Italy. As the Europeans developed the New World, they brought sugarcane, presses, and slaves with them to produce sugar and rum. By 1550, 3,000 sugar mills blanketed Brazil and the rest of South America. In 1625, sugar production spread to the Caribbean islands including Jamaica, Haiti, and Cuba. The need for cast-iron equipment to build and maintain these mills helped spark Europe's industrial revolution.[22] Increasing mechanization of sugarcane harvesting and sugar production led to sharply lower prices. This gave access to sugar to a growing worldwide population with a serious sweet tooth. Sugar consumption in Britain rose from 18 pounds per person per year in 1700 to 100 pounds by the end of the 20th century.

In 1747, sucrose was discovered in beet root, and the first sugar beet factory opened in Poland in 1801. Cut off from the Caribbean sugar supplies by the British blockade in 1813, Napoleon instituted a ban on sugar imports, a move that quickly grew the mechanized beet sugar industry. By 1837, there were 542 sugar beet factories in France alone. While it was slow to take off in North America, sugar beet farming now makes up 55 percent of the 8.1 million tons of sugar produced every year in the United States. Beet sugar isn't the only sweetener to compete for our affections. When sugar prices spiked in the United States in the late 1970s and early 1980s due to import quotas and tariffs, much cheaper high-fructose corn syrup quickly replaced cane sugar in processed foods and soft drinks. Sugar consumption in the United States hit its peak in 1999 with Americans consuming

111 grams of sugar per day. In 2015, we slurped down 94 grams of sugar daily, the majority blended discretely into sweet drinks and processed foods.[23]

**HOW MUCH SUGAR DO YOU HAVE IN YOUR BODY?**

Glucose is a critical part of our cellular metabolism and design. The human body contains about 4 pounds of sugar. Sweet.

The sugar wars started in response to our old friend Ancel Keys' first attacks on saturated fats as the cause of heart disease. John Yudkin, a London physiologist, took a contrarian view that sugar was the culprit. Two decades of sparring between the well-funded camps ensued, culminating in Yudkin's popular 1972 book, *Pure, White, and Deadly: The Problem of Sugar*.[24] Despite a dearth of evidence, the popular backlash was so strong that when the McGovern report was published in 1977, it recommended a 40 percent cut in national sugar consumption.

In 2016, world production of sugar reached nearly 180 million tons. Granted, some of that goes to make ethanol for our cars and alcohol for our weekends, but it's still a ridiculous amount. Although Americans consume about 25 percent less sugar per year than the British did a century ago, sugar is blamed by some health advocates for the spread of type 2 diabetes, heart disease, arthritis, and cancer. In his 2016 book, *The Case against Sugar*, science journalist Gary Taubes channeled his inner Yudkin and argues that sugar should be treated as an illegal drug because it is the primary cause for most disease.[25] Discounting the effects of overeating, smoking, sedentary living, and obesity, he weaves a tale that equates table sugar to cocaine and an FDA trapped in the pockets of malevolent scientists and Big Sugar special interests. While it is true that sugar is often added to tobacco during processing, sugar is not cigarette smoking.

Taubes believes that scientists overly complicate research and that sugar triggers insulin resistance, obesity, diabetes, Alzheimer's disease, gout, and heart disease. But if sugar consumption has declined since 1999, why have obesity and diabetes increased?[26, 27] We already know that insulin resistance can accelerate aging and metabolic disease. Insulin resistance does not cause obesity. Obesity and physical inactivity *cause* insulin resistance.[28, 29] A 2017 study found that obesity leads to inflammatory changes and induction of interleukin-32 (IL-32), a potent myogenic regulator.[30] IL-32 creates methylation changes in the DNA muscle stem cells that shut down development and their substitution in muscle by adipose. Fat breeding fat.

Taubes thinks that the fructose in table sugar (a disaccharide consisting of 55 percent fructose and 45 percent sucrose) ruins the liver, leading to insulin resistance that causes obesity. The problem is that is not how your body works. Fructose can screw up your liver, but only when your liver energy storage capacity is already full and you overeat on a high-fat, high-fructose diet.[31] This leads to high levels of fructokinase enzyme activity and ATP depletion. Listen up, even though I'm saying that sugar does not cause insulin resistance or obesity, if you're already fat and diabetic, you should limit the sugar in your diet. I know, another medical shocker.

Pay close attention. Even though fat and sugar by themselves are not necessarily threatening, they do make very bad bedfellows. If you continually overeat on a high-carbohydrate, high-fat diet, you will get liver disease.[32] You also have to keep in mind that your genome is very sensitive to diet. These changes are particularly pronounced early in life, so that while an adult might be able to tolerate long stretches of a high-fat or high-carbohydrate diet and emerge unscathed, the same may not be true for children. A study in flies, who love sugar even more than we do, found long-term changes in gene expression and a 7 percent shorter life span when they were fed a sugar-dense diet early in life.[33]

The real menace is obesity. A study by the National Institutes of Health in 2014 found that extreme obesity can shorten your life by as much as 14 years.[34] Obesity increases your risk of dying early in many fundamental ways. It can cause insulin resistance and accelerate aging via metabolic channels. It can also cause cancer. When you become obese, your pancreas produces more proteolytic enzymes like chymotrypsin.[35] If it reaches high levels, this serine protease depletes your intestinal cells of natural tumor suppressor receptors like neogenin and DCC (Deleted in Colorectal Cancer) that would normally kill potential cancer cells. Way not cool.

Obesity can also fry your motherboard. High caloric intake and obesity have been associated with dementia, cognitive impairment, and Alzheimer's disease.[36] The reasons behind this may be hidden in our DNA. The brain has proteins called apolipoproteins that bind fat and cholesterol to transport them to the lymphatic system for disposal. A 2017 study on mice has shown that obesity can trigger Alzheimer's disease when the fat rats have an inflammatory-producing version of the apolipoprotein gene called ApoE4, instead of the more common ApoE3 version.[37]

## EVEN BETTER THAN THE REAL THING

Artificial sweeteners are an eclectic group used throughout the United States and the world as zero- or low-calorie alternatives to sugar for use in beverages and food. Most are hundreds of times sweeter than sugar. Even as the consumption of sodas has decreased over the past 20 years, the use of sugar substitutes has been rising.

Originally meant to replace sugar in sweetened beverages and foods for diabetic patients and obese patients trying to lose weight, artificial sweeteners have always had unintended consequences. The first artificial sweetener was lead acetate (lead sugar). It was first used by the Romans, who boiled wine in lead pots to create a distillate called *sapa* that was used as an alternative to honey to sweeten wine and preserve fruits. Later, lead sugar was produced by treating lead oxidized with acetic acid to form a water-soluble, mildly sweet, white crystalline powder used for medicinal purposes. Although its use as a food additive faded as the toxicity of lead became acknowledged, lead acetate was used in cosmetics until 2004 and is still used in hair coloring treatments today (I'm looking at you, Grecian Formula).

Like most sugar substitutes, saccharin was discovered by scientists tasting strange new compounds. Apparently, chemists can't keep their fingers out of their mouths. The first contemporary artificial sweetener, saccharin is 300 to 400 times sweeter than sucrose and was produced by scientists in 1879 while working on coal tar derivatives for paint thinners. It was introduced in the United States at the turn of the century and became popular in Europe during the sugar shortages caused by World War I. Concerns over possible cancer links appeared in animal studies during the 1970s, leading to FDA-mandated package warnings. The warning labels were dropped in 2001, after human studies failed to confirm these cancer concerns. Saccharin is the main component of the table sweetener Sweet-N-Low, where it is cut with dextrose to dull its sweetness for consumer use.

The weakest, cheapest, and most maligned of all sugar replacements is sodium cyclamate. It was accidently created in 1935 by a grad student at the University of Illinois, named Michael Sveda, while he was working on developing anti-fever pills. No, he didn't stick a contaminated finger in his mouth. This time it was a cigarette he left lying on his lab bench in some cyclamate residue. *I wonder why this cig tastes so damn good?* Nice technique, Mike. Because they are much more heat stable than other sugar substitutes, cyclamates quickly found their way into the kitchen. By 1969, cyclamates were crushing it with annual sales exceeding $1 billion. Their fall from grace was epic. Researchers reported they caused bladder cancer in animals. Although the reports were never confirmed in humans, cyclamates were flogged in the press and finally banned in the United States in 1970. Despite the failure of long-term studies to prove that cyclamates are carcinogenic, the ban remains in place. Outside the United States, however, cyclamates remain in heavy use.

Another popular sugar substitute is aspartame, a non-saccharin-based compound that is 200 times sweeter than sucrose. It was accidently discovered in 1965 (back to the finger thing) during the pharmaceutical development of a hormone-based drug to prevent ulcers. Aspartame also had a rocky road to FDA approval, with unconfirmed concerns over possible brain cancer links. It was first approved for carbonated beverages, but was not given full US clearance until 1996. Because aspartame hydrolyzes quickly during digestion to aspartic acid, phenylalanine, and methanol, people with the rare inherited metabolic disorder phenylketonuria should not consume anything containing aspartame. You know aspartame as Equal or NutraSweet, and it is now the most popular sugar substitute in the world, used in more than 6,000 products worldwide.

The newest and sweetest (600 times as sweet as sucrose) modern sugar-free compound is sucralose. Discovered in 1976 by chemists chlorinating sucrose to try to make an insecticide, sucralose is so sweet that it gets cut 99:1 with dextrose to make it acceptable for table use in products like Splenda.

Even if we set aside 60 years of inconclusive data linking artificial sweeteners to cancer, we still have one problem. They don't work. Oh, they're sweet and we really, really like them, but they aren't going to help you lose weight or live longer. In fact, there is mounting data that habitual use of diet sodas containing artificial sweeteners *causes* obesity and increased blood sugar levels.[38, 39] In 2014, immunologists found mice fed saccharin, aspartame, or sucralose all developed alterations in their gut microflora followed by glucose intolerance.[40] How does this work? If our gut bacteria population shifts, it changes how we extract nutrients during digestion, and this can cause metabolic disease. The researchers found humans developed similar changes in gut bacteria and glucose tolerance after drinking sugar-substitute drinks after only a week.

The case against sugar substitutes gets stronger every year. In 2017, data from the long-term Framingham heart study linked the consumption of *artificially* sweetened beverages with increased risks of stroke and dementia.[41, 42] In contrast, the same study also concluded that *naturally* sugar-sweetened beverages did not increase the risk of stroke or dementia.

What do you do now? Is sugar good for you? Not particularly, but if you can keep a lid on the tin, real sugar is still *way* better than all this rebadged lab waste. You still have to watch the processed foods. Heck, they even sneak some sugar into my Bordeaux. What's with that? With all the doubts about sugar and artificial sweeteners, attention has been turned to other naturally based sugar substitutes, like stevia (the plant, not Wonder). The *Stevia rebaudiana* plant has been in use for more than 1,500 years in South America. The leaves are sweet because they contain steviol glycosides (200 times sweeter than sugar), and they have a licorice aftertaste. Stevia was first introduced as a commercial sweetener in Japan and now holds a 40 percent market share there. It found its way into the United States as an herbal food additive in the 1980s, but it was banned by the FDA in 1991 after early studies considered it possibly carcinogenic. In 2008, the FDA allowed some stevia extracts, like rebaudioside A, into the US market. Now available as Truvia (Coca-Cola) and PureVia (PepsiCo), these preparations bear little resemblance to native stevia. The production of rebiana from the stevia herb is a complicated 40-step chemical refining process using acetone and other wholesome pharmaceuticals. Distilled rebiana is intense stuff. It's so harshly sweet that a packet of Truvia or PureVia contains only 0.05 percent rebiana and 99.5 percent erythritol. Talk about raw. But, hey, it's natural, so it must be good for you.

## THE MAN TRAP

I love watching the old *Star Trek* television show. My favorite episode of all time is when James Tiberius Kirk battles a hungry salt-monster. His best bud, Bones, the ship's doctor, is seduced and drugged by a sodium-craving, shape-shifting succubus posing as his old flame. After a bug hunt that goes on way too long, Kirk outs the beast after she gets the drop on him and his Vulcan sidekick, Spock. Luckily, Bones snaps out of his trance just in time to give the creature a face full of phaser before she drains the captain of all his saline. Trust me, it's precious stuff. It wasn't Bill Shatner's fault, but ever since then, I've had serious issues with salt.

Dietary salt (about 40 percent sodium) has been demonized by medicine and politicians for more than 100 years.[43] Despite the absence of any meaningful data, we've been told that a high salt intake causes high blood pressure, which leads to a stroke and an exit even earlier than a *Star Trek* crewman in a red shirt. This has created huge problems because humans love salt as much as we love sugar. And that's okay, because, like fat and sugar, we all respond differently to salt. Remember, we are the masters of metabolic flexibility and our kidneys evolved to regulate a broad range of salinity.

Over the past few years, an increasing amount of solid research has questioned the tenuous connection between salt and high blood pressure. A review of prospective (i.e., good) studies in 2011 found minimal improvements in blood pressure with salt restriction and no effect on cardiovascular events.[44] In 2014, a study in the *New England Journal of Medicine* found that people who consumed a moderate amount of salt per day (3 to 6 grams/day) had fewer cardiac events than people who had large (>6 grams/day) or small amounts (<3 grams/day) of daily salt intake.[45] In a large, well-designed French study also published in 2014, researchers found no direct connection between salt intake and hypertension.[46] They did find that some people appear to be very sensitive to salt, but concluded that obesity was the primary cause of hypertension in their study. In 2017, a study of 130,00 people from 49 nations found that while high salt intake should be discouraged in patients who already have hypertension (about 10 percent of study participants), salt-restricted diets *increased* the rates of heart attacks, strokes, and deaths compared to those people with average salt intake.[47]

Intriguing data collected during isolation testing for deep space missions undermines one of the oldest-held nutritional beliefs: salt makes you thirsty.[48] When fed high-salt diets, the captive cosmonauts shed higher amounts of salt in their urine, but they drank much less. It turns out that even though they made more urine, they still maintained a constant level of sodium in their blood. How? They made more glucocorticoids. These steroids break down tissue in the muscle and liver to make urea. It seems that urea isn't just a nitrogen wastebasket; it's a powerful, potentially life-saving osmolyte that links salt intake to metabolic balance. Animal studies have previously also shown increased urea production with hikes in dietary salt. Both mice and men were hungrier and ate more when their salt intakes were high. Scientists believe this may be driven by the spike in energy consumption needed to mobilize nitrogen and produce urea and water to dilute sodium in the bloodstream.[49] Surprise, salt makes you hungry, not thirsty. If you think that just skipping the saltshaker will make you thinner, it is important to realize that 75 percent of the salt we consume is hidden in processed and prepared food.

High salt intake can also foment a revolution in your gut microflora. Increased salinity in your stomach can increase the production of harmful enzymes by bacteria.[50] One of these proteases, subtilisin, is like chymotrypsin and can cause chronic inflammation and cancer. The induction of subtilisin by a high-salt diet might be one of the reasons that stomach cancer is so common among middle-aged Japanese.[51] Sounds terrible.

Why not just cut salt out completely? Granted, it makes all my boring, healthy foods taste a little better, but it also provides a delivery route for something our bodies need way more—iodine. Global iodine deficiency is a serious problem. According to the World Health Organization, nearly two billion people worldwide are iodine deficient. More than 187 million have thyroid problems like goiter, neurologic damage, and hypothyroidism, which hammers their metabolism. Seafood is an important dietary source of iodine but is not accessible for large swaths of the populations. Salt iodization with potassium iodate has been adopted in many developing countries to address this. No monster necessary.

## ORTHOREXIA GLUTENOSA

Orthorexia nervosa is not some exotic bone disorder that wrecks your nervous system; it's an actual medical condition marked by an unhealthy, obsessive need to avoid foods thought to be unhealthy. It is an eating disorder of exclusion. The newest addition to orthorexia's hit list is a familiar name: wheat. Domesticated as a crop since 9600 BC, wheat is second only to maize in world production at more than 740 million tons per year. Wheat contains carbohydrates, fiber, and protein. It's one of these binding proteins, gluten, that has become a lightning rod for concern over the past 5 years. Gluten is a biocomposite made up of sticky proteins called prolamins and glutelins that helps trap carbon dioxide and water during fermentation. This helps bread and pastry to rise and gives it a springy, elastic quality. Gluten is found in many types of both natural and processed foods, including garlic, soy sauce, and beer, making it one of the most heavily consumed proteins on the planet. Because it makes for a very efficient binding agent, gluten is also used in making cosmetics, hair products, and moisturizing creams.

Approximately 0.7 percent of the US population has a genetically mediated autoimmune disorder called celiac disease. People with true celiac disease display a violent immunologic reaction to even a trace amount of gluten in any form, developing severe small intestinal inflammation and damage that wrecks normal nutrient absorption.[52] The mechanisms underlying celiac disease are unclear, but researchers suspect

**DANGERS OF A G-FREE LIFE**

If you substitute rice flour for wheat in a gluten-free diet, you run the risk of accumulating some nasty toxins. Mercury, cadmium, and arsenic poisons stick to rice like glue and can build up in your tissues. Going r-free might be better.

that dormant, inherited celiac genes buried in the DNA are activated by gluten or other environmental triggers. Celiac patients have a radically altered microbiome, and the role of gut bacteria in the disease is being heavily investigated. Research is focused on developing immunotherapy to treat celiac disease, but for now the only treatment is to be zealously gluten-free. Even when completely gluten-free, celiac patients can still develop inflammatory and metabolic disorders like diabetes, arthritis, and osteoporosis.

Although celiac disease is uncommon, there are indications that the number of full-blown celiacs may be increasing along with a growing number of people who have gluten or wheat sensitivity. Some researchers believe that this is because we are consuming wheat and gluten-based food at historic levels. The problem is that we are not. Yes, we love our bread here in the States, but we used to love it even more. Way more. In 1900, wheat consumption (code for gluten) peaked at around 220 pounds per year per person.[53] That's a lot of dough, baby. In contrast, we buttered up only 110 pounds of the chewy stuff in 1970 and toasted up 134 pounds in 2008. So, no, we're not eating more wheat today. I say this at the same time I am eyeballing a seriously delicious-looking pizza commercial. Sorry, I am easily distracted.

There is also a presumption that if the sheer tonnage of wheat consumed per year is not the reason for the obesity epidemic and widespread gastric mayhem, then the culprit must be our modern, genetically modified *Franken-wheat*. Your honor, I object. A careful comparative analysis of contemporary wheat cultivars showed no change in relative gluten content over the past century.[54] As for obesity, you know where I stand. High-carbohydrate (bread, etc.) diets do not cause obesity. Hypercaloric consumption does.

In the wake of popular health and diet books like David Perlmutter's *Grain Brain: The Surprising Truth about Wheat, Carbs, and Sugar—Your Brain's Silent Killers* that extol the harmful effects of whole grains and the virtues of a life without wheat, many people have adopted a grain-free lifestyle.[55] In 2015, an estimated 25 percent of Americans bought gluten-free food, a 67 percent jump from 2013. Gluten-free is now very big business. Global gluten-free food sales jumped 12.6 percent in 2016 to $3.5 billion and have doubled in only 8 years.

Isn't a gluten-free diet better for you? Not necessarily. Diets containing carbohydrates rich in gluten have never been associated with obesity, cardiovascular disease, or metabolic disease in non-celiac patients. Even claims of elevated blood sugars and sky-high glycemic indices don't ring true. Everyone reacts differently to the same dietary blend of carbohydrates.[56, 57] This is because the trillions of bacteria that line our gut determine how much glucose we can absorb from our food, and this population mix varies from person to person. Because of this, the traditional use of glycemic indices to design diets is unreliable.

But what about people who don't have celiac disease but have a self-diagnosed gluten sensitivity? There must be a lot of them getting sick from this silent threat. Right? Wrong. A blinded experiment was conducted to find out if they could tell if they were eating gluten or not. It turns out that they can't tell the difference.[58] Even after removing potentially gassy FODMAPS (an acronym for fructans and other short-chain carbs that aren't absorbed during digestion), the self-diagnosed gluten-sensitive couldn't perceive a difference between food with or without it.[59]

The biggest lie about gluten-free diets is that they are healthier for you. Gluten does not cause cardiovascular disease, and being gluten-free will not help you live longer.[60] Then there is the whole toxic metal thing. The what?

Most commercial gluten-free food uses rice flour as a substitute for wheat flour to improve its taste and consistency. The problem is that rice is one of the world's biggest dietary sources of carcinogenic arsenic and methylmercury. Rice is like a poison sponge. A recent study of patients on a gluten-free diet found elevated levels of these nasty toxins in the blood and urine.[61] Yikes. I plan on keeping pizza in my life a little longer and skipping the whole gluten-free thing.

## THE SWEET SPOT

Fat, salt, sugar, and gluten. Stop obsessing about every little macronutrient in your diet. Trust me, it will make your next trip to Stop and Shop a lot less stressful. But what about all the diet recommendations you see headlined on the news every night? Anyone who has ever watched a disaster movie epic knows that it takes a long time for scientists to change their opinions. Despite 4 decades of research to the contrary, most Western governments still promote the position that saturated fat causes heart disease rather than the fact that the main cause is overeating. The unintended consequence of recommending decreased intake of saturated fats is their blind substitution by many people with nutritionally low-value carbohydrates.

There are signs that the dietary guideline tides finally may be shifting. One of the largest prospective diet studies ever undertaken questions traditional food advice. The Prospective Urban Rural Epidemiology (PURE) study from McMaster University is a massive undertaking by any standards.[62, 63] The PURE study is a logistic wonder. A truly global project, it surveyed 135,000 people from 18 countries across five continents and a broad socioeconomic range. New data from PURE suggests that a diet with saturated fat and a reasonable amount of carbs had the best mortality rate. In fact, dietary fats had no effect on the incidence of cardiovascular disease or heart attacks. None. So much for the diet-heart hypothesis. In fact, those people who ate a low-fat diet did the worst, dying prematurely at a 13 percent higher rate, while people eating a diet relatively high in saturated fat had less risk of stroke and a 23 percent lower mortality rate. Mortality rates were highest in those who got more than 60 percent of their daily calories from carbohydrates.

The recommendation from PURE researchers is to shoot for 50 to 55 percent of calories from carbohydrates and 35 percent from a mix of saturated and unsaturated fats. Hard to argue with those numbers. One caveat: Because the PURE study is observational, we have to be careful interpreting the data. Nonetheless, its lack of support for the hypothesis that dietary fat causes heart disease is striking.

Can you knock down an occasional duo of chili-doused, cheese-drenched bacon burgers and still survive? Yes. Should you? Come on, man, moderation is the key. Each of us responds differently to different diets, and, if we don't abuse it, metabolic durability will continue to be our greatest survival advantage individually and as a species. As long as you stick to a generally plant-based diet, keep the carbs around the caloric halfway mark, and don't go Neanderthal on your protein consumption, you'll be fine. Did someone say protein? Yes, I'm coming for you contemporary cavemen next.

# DIET'S MOST WANTED LIST

Vilified, hunted, and excluded, most of these nutritional suspects are accused of crimes they never committed.

## SATURATED FAT

Fat does not cause heart disease. Inflammation does. You need cholesterol to make hormones and cell membranes.

**1**

## SUGAR

**2**

Sugar does not cause diabetes. Obesity and a burned-out pancreas do. Avoid eating processed food and adding sugar.

## SALT

Salt will make you hungry, but it won't give you high blood pressure. Obesity does.

**3**

## GLUTEN

**4**

Unless you have celiac disease or a documented gluten allergy, relax. There are bigger bears in this forest.

## SUGAR SUBSTITUTES

Guilty as charged. Aspartame, saccharin, and sucralose are awful things and terrible for your health.

**5**

### FOOD IS NOT THE ENEMY.

# 7

# A HIGH-STEAKS GAME

**THERE ARE THREE MAIN** macronutrients in all diets: protein, carbohydrates, and fat. The current adult dietary guidelines from the National Institutes of Health recommend 10 to 35 percent of total energy from protein, 45 to 65 percent from carbohydrates, and 20 to 35 percent from fat.[1] Proteins are made up of long chains of amino acids called polypeptides. Our bodies use amino acids to build proteins to build, maintain, and repair tissue. Proteins and their 20 component amino acids present a dilemma for the body. Unlike plants, we can't make them all and have no way to store the leftovers for later use.

Our bodies can synthesize what are called *nonessential amino acids:* alanine, asparagine, aspartic acid, cysteine, glutamic acid, glutamine, serine, proline, glycine, and tyrosine (made from phenylalanine). The rest are called *essential amino acids,* and we can get them only from our diet: arginine, histidine, isoleucine, leucine, lysine, methionine, valine, tryptophan, phenylalanine, and valine. Hey, I have 10 brothers- and sisters-in-law; you can handle 10 essential amino acids.

We need some dietary protein to survive, but how much? The current recommended daily amount is 0.8 grams of protein per kilogram of body weight. That translates to a paltry 46 grams per day for the average woman and 56 grams per day for a man. Most Americans consume way more protein than this *at every meal.* Daily protein consumption in the United States has been hovering around 100 grams per day since 1909.[2, 3] Athletes eat even more; many get most of their calories from protein while training. Diets super high in protein and low in carbohydrates, like the Paleo Diet, Atkins Diet, and Whole30, have become popular because of the widely held belief that they are healthy and promote weight loss.[4, 5, 6] Evangelistic supporters of Big Protein cite higher satiety, higher metabolic rates, increased strength, weight loss, and improved energy after only a few days of starting. Sounds too good to be true. And it is.

## WHERE'S THE BEEF?

The amount of energy (calories) you burn every day is made up of three parts: baseline metabolic rate, physical activity, and the energy used to metabolize the food you eat. This third component is also called diet-induced thermogenesis (DIT), a function of the caloric content of the food and how much energy is needed to metabolize it.[7] In general, DIT is highest for alcohol, followed by protein, carbohydrates, and fat. The overall DIT for a standard diet is between 5 and 15 percent of total energy expenditure. Theoretically, if you ate a diet very high in protein and low in fat, you would burn more calories eating the same amount of food. Some researchers also believe that high-protein diets with high DIT produce less hunger and are easier to maintain.[8] Since protein has the same calorie value as carbohydrate (4 calories per gram) and much less than fat (9 calories per gram), high-protein diets will produce rapid weight loss.

All these things are true, but this way of thinking is a trap. A big, juicy, medium-rare, meaty trap. Our bodies have evolved to maintain a steady energy state for survival. We use our innate superpower of metabolic flexibility to adapt to a wide range of food sources and supply. Bottom line, high-protein diets fool the body for only a little while before it resets the energy balance thermostat. Any minor caloric or satiety advantage from protein quickly evaporates.

## WHEY TO GO

There is a reason it takes more energy to break down proteins. It's hard on the body. When protein is metabolized into circulating amino acids, your blood becomes, wait for it . . . a little more acidic. To balance this out and keep your pH steady at the slightly alkaline sweet spot of 7.4, the body needs a base. Normally our lungs (carbon dioxide) and kidneys (ammonium) can handle small buffering loads. However, high-protein diets produce large amounts of amino acids that stress pH balance mechanisms. You would have to eat a ridiculous amount of vegetables to neutralize all that acid. What does the body use to balance the pH? Calcium. The source of all this extra calcium is hotly debated. Some scientists believe it comes from increased intestinal dietary absorption. Others think it comes from excavation of our biggest reservoir of calcium, the skeleton, and that it is a major cause of osteoporosis.[9]

In either case, the waste calcium phosphate, carbonate, and ammonium is flushed out of the body in the urine. Since we don't store excess amino acid that we don't use, excess nitrogen waste is also filtered through the kidneys. High-protein diets stress the kidneys by increasing glomerular filtration rates. This leads to a whole lot of peeing. To avoid dehydration and possible stone formation (ouch), you need to drink a lot more water. Which leads to more peeing. In a healthy young kidney, this is usually handled well, but if you're older or have any renal issues, high-protein diets can absolutely wreck the beans. Maybe the weight loss comes from all those desperate bathroom runs.

# MISSING LINKS

Even if high-protein diets did help you lose a little weight or feel a little more vital, they still have one big problem. They can kill you. Frank Hu and his team at the Harvard School of Public Health measured the animal and plant protein intakes of 131,342 participants in the Nurses' Health and Health Professionals Follow-Up Studies.[10] They found high animal protein consumption in people who had a defined lifestyle risk factor (obesity, inactivity, smoking, or alcohol use) was associated with cardiovascular mortality. Those that had high plant protein intake had lower risk of death from heart disease. Another long-term study of 536,000 men and women ages 50 to 71 found that those with the diets highest in red and processed meat had a 26 percent higher risk of dying from heart disease, cancer, stroke, diabetes, infections, lung disease, and kidney disease than those with the lowest. The authors suggest that iron in hemoglobin from red meat and the nitrates/nitrites used in processing might be the cause of the higher death rates. This conclusion is also supported by their additional finding that participants who ate higher levels of fish and poultry had a 25 percent lower risk of dying from these causes than those who consumed lower amounts.[11] These findings are consistent with a 2016 study that found a 59 percent higher all-cause mortality rate in people who ate a high protein intake diet compared to the low-pro folks.[12]

If that's not enough to get you to cancel your porterhouse power lunch reservation, it gets worse. It turns out that eating a high-protein diet during middle age can be even more toxic than smoking. Why? Once again, the reasons can be traced to metabolism. It is well known that high-protein diets trigger elevation of insulin growth factor-1 (IGF-1). This was initially thought to be a good thing, since IGF-1 was believed to help build stronger bones. Well, like a lot of stuff in science, the more we look at something, the worse it begins to look. There is a remote village in Ecuador where residents have a genetic disorder that mutates their growth hormone receptor (GHR) gene, leading to severe GHR and IGF-1 deficiencies. This disorder, called Laron syndrome, causes dwarfism and obesity, but the mutation eliminates the age-related diseases of cancer and diabetes. If they didn't have Laron syndrome, these villagers would normally have a 17 percent cancer and a 5 percent diabetes rate.

Jaime Guevara-Aguirre and Valter Longo's lab at the University of Southern California studied blood samples from the GHR/IGF-1 deficient villagers.[13] They had low insulin levels and low insulin resistance, possibly explaining their failure to develop diabetes. Next, the researchers took

> **PALEO PROBLEMS**
>
> A diet high in protein is a high-risk proposition as you get older. It can overload your kidneys, thin your bones, and promote cancer. There's a reason the Neanderthals are extinct.

typical stock human skin cell samples and injected them with hydrogen GHR/IGF-1 deficient serum. Remarkably, the damaged cells showed signs of healing, with increased apoptosis and antioxidant levels, and decreased precancerous proteins (Ras) and the aging accelerant mTOR (mechanistic target of rapamycin).

That's some pretty good work. But Longo and his team kicked it up a notch in a 2014 follow-up study examining the relationship between non-plant-based protein intake and death in older people.[14] They surveyed 6,381 American men and women over the age of 50. The respondents were then divided into three groups defined by their protein consumption—high (20 percent total calorie intake from protein), moderate (10 to 19 percent), and low (<10 percent). They were then followed prospectively for 18 years. People with high protein intake didn't make out so well. They had a 73 times increased risk of diabetes mortality. High protein intake participants between ages 50 and 65 had a 74 percent higher risk of death from all causes and a 4 times higher risk of dying from cancer. The moderate protein intake group had a 23 times increase in diabetic mortality and a 3 times higher risk of dying from cancer. Low protein and plant-based protein intake did not correlate with increased death rates. People over 65 did way better with high protein intake, and this group had a little lower mortality and cancer rate, perhaps because protein absorption decreases after the age of 70.

Longo and his group then went further. They randomly tested IGF-1 levels in one-third of the study respondents and found that IGF-1 correlated well with protein intake under age 65. Higher protein intake, higher IGF-1. When they matched this up against death rates, the results were sobering. For every 10 milligrams/milliliter increase in IGF-1, the risk of dying from cancer rises 9 percent. Still not convinced? Neither were they. They added a series of experiments to confirm the high protein/death link. First, they exposed yeast cells to increasingly higher concentrations of amino acids. The result? As the unicellular organisms aged (apparently, 5 days old is middle aged for a yeast), they showed increasing DNA mutation rates and genomic instability as amino acid exposure increased.

Next, they moved to mammals. Mice fed a high-protein chow had IGF-1 levels 35 percent higher than the furry guys on low-protein food. IGF-1 binding protein levels were very high in the low-protein group and may be the reason circulating levels of IGF-1 were lower in this group. When they implanted these unlucky rodents with tumor cells, the mice on high-protein diets had their tumors progress 78 percent faster than the low-pro mice. The researchers wanted even more proof, so they implanted similar tumors into mice engineered to be GHR/IGF-1 deficient. No tumor growth. Touchdown.

That is one badass experiment. The conclusions are clear. High-protein diets in people under 65 are linked to diabetes, cancer, and early death. The mechanism appears to be a double whammy of DNA damage and metabolic mayhem mediated by insulin growth factor. No bacon slice is worth that.

A diet high in red meat can also cause cancer through another, even sneakier, route: hijacking your own microflora. Depending on your microbial signature, a diet heavy on red meat can result in your bacteria producing potentially toxic and carcinogenic substances like deoxycholic acid (colon cancer), 2-amino-1-methyl-6-phenylimidazo-[4,5-b]-pyridine (PhIP) (prostate cancer), and trimethyl-$N$-amine oxide (TMO) (colorectal cancer).[15] Bacillus bacteria also produce a ruthless little enzyme called subtilisin that is used as a meat tenderizer as well as many other things, including detergents and solvents. It causes chronic systemic inflammation and could be another factor linking diet, environment, and cancer. There is some evidence that compounds called Bowman-Birk factors can inhibit the effects of subtilisin and chymotrypsin to reduce their carcinogenic effects. These serine protease inhibitors are produced by many plants, including potatoes, wheat, lentils, and soy, and can reduce the potential carcinogenic effects of meat.

## CAVEAT MTOR

Nutritional science has always been considered a little "soft" by other disciplines. The main problem is that they deal with a myriad of diet factors in often uncontrolled environments. Add to this the most unpredictable element of all, the subject, and it makes the application of rigorous scientific method challenging. Enter the Geometric Framework for Nutrition. It's a space model that allows very precise measurement of the impact of complex nutritional elements on health. Using the Geometric Framework, a group from the University of Sydney has made the most ambitious attempt yet to assess the impact of macronutrient intake on health, disease, and longevity.[16] They assessed 25 different diet blends and caloric amounts of protein, carbohydrates, and fat on freely fed mice. When concentrations of protein or carbohydrates were decreased, the mice ate more. Mice lived the longest (30 percent longer) when the blend was lowest in protein and highest in carbohydrate. These guys also had much better overall health indices: lower blood pressure, better glucose tolerance, higher high-density lipoprotein, lower low-density lipoprotein, and lower triglycerides.

The researchers found liver mTOR levels rose as the protein-to-carbohydrate ratio increased in the Geometric Framework diet test blends. When you are young and growing, packing some heavy mTOR is fine. It helps coordinate metabolism with amino acid supplies, insulin levels, and energy supplies, and it promotes growth. As you get older, however, high levels of mTOR are a very, very bad thing. High mTOR disrupts the metabolic balance of an organism in a fundamental and pervasive way. It drains your precious ATP energy reserves by hijacking phosphate ions and throwing them around your system like a drunk with a checkbook. It makes bad things, like cancer, grow- and allows disease to progress as it disrupts crucial autophagic recycling pathways and apoptosis. Plasma free amino acids, especially the branched chain kind, along with IGF-1, rise with protein intake and trigger mTOR. This is the main reason why there is so much interest in drugs that could quench mTOR to improve health and longevity. (We'll discuss this further in Chapter 16.)

For the young and growing, diets high in protein make some sense. You need to build bone and muscle tissue, and those nimble young kidneys can handle the extra flow rate and nitrogen filtration load. After the age of 50, it's very different story. Throttle back on the red meat and dial up the carbs to keep your energy levels high and mortality risk low. You don't need the extra renal stress or genomic instability. For most of us, that means a ruthless 50 percent cut in our total protein (both plant and animal) intake every day. And lots of vegetables on the side to break down those serine proteases and buffer the pH levels. I don't know about you, but if it keeps my DNA from looking like a game of Battleship, I'm totally in. Don't worry, I'll be back wrapping my steak in bacon again after I hit 70, when I'll need some meat on my bones.

Now that we've seen the good, bad, and downright ugly of the American Way, it's time to have a go at the flipside. Release the Vegan.

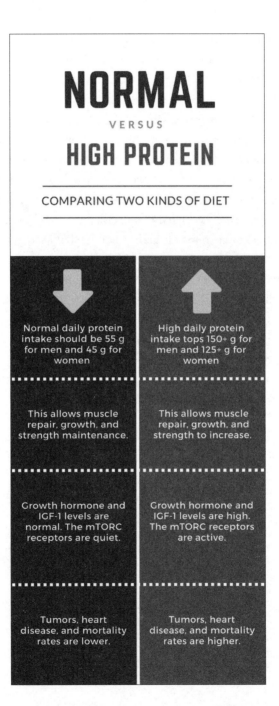

# NORMAL

VERSUS

# HIGH PROTEIN

COMPARING TWO KINDS OF DIET

| Normal daily protein intake should be 55 g for men and 45 g for women | High daily protein intake tops 150+ g for men and 125+ g for women |
|---|---|
| This allows muscle repair, growth, and strength maintenance. | This allows muscle repair, growth, and strength to increase. |
| Growth hormone and IGF-1 levels are normal. The mTORC receptors are quiet. | Growth hormone and IGF-1 levels are high. The mTORC receptors are active. |
| Tumors, heart disease, and mortality rates are lower. | Tumors, heart disease, and mortality rates are higher. |

# 8

# GREEN IS THE NEW BLACK

"A mind of the caliber of mine cannot derive its nutriment from cows."

—GEORGE BERNARD SHAW,1890

VEGAN, VEGETARIAN, LACTO-VEGETARIAN, OVO vegetarian, lacto-ovo vegetarian, pescatarian, lacto-ovo pescatarian—whatever the label, few issues inspire more passionate debate than the decision to not eat meat. I know it's confusing. Even vegetarians muddy the waters by varying their diets by time and date. For the record, vegans are hard-core—no animal stuff at all, no refined products, and no animal-tested products. After that it's a free-for-all. Vegetarians as groups do not eat meat, though some will eat dairy products but not eggs (lacto-vegetarians); others will eat eggs but not dairy (ovo vegetarians); some eat both dairy and eggs (lacto-ovo vegetarians); and many will eat fish and/or shellfish (pesco-vegetarian/seagan). Are they even vegetarian? Some forms of vegetarianism exclude certain vegetables, and many won't eat honey. But some vegans eat honey. Buddhist vegetarians (as well as many self-identified vegetarians) will even eat meat. It's enough to make your head explode.

The reasons for going *sin carne* freely cross borders of health, religion, environment, ethics, morality, and even politics. Despite the rising popularity of vegetarian restaurants and increasing cultural acceptance in the United States (or is it just Manhattan?), a poll from the Vegetarian Resource Group in 2016 found only 3.3 percent of Americans are vegetarian, and of those, 1.6 percent are full-on, dairy-free vegans. The same poll also noted vegetarian/vegan diets are much more popular among younger rather than older Americans (5.3 percent of people ages 18 to 34 versus 1.8 percent of people over the age of 65).[1] A poll from the Humane Resource Council (Faunalytics.org) of 11,000 Americans found that while 12 percent had tried vegetarian diets, only one of five could maintain it, and 84 percent gave it up altogether to go back to eating meat.[2] Most vegetarians are women, with 74 percent identifying as female, compared to 51 percent in the general population.

Vegetarianism dates back as early as 7000 BC during the Bronze Age and was used for medical and religious practices in Egypt. It spread as a religious movement through ancient Greece led by the philosophers Pythagoras, Seneca, and Plutarch. Vegetarianism continued to prosper during the early Roman Empire, but faded following its Christianization. In India, vegetarianism found some synergism with Hinduism and thrived there during the Middle Ages. Vegetarianism returned to Europe during the Renaissance as a more secular, ethical practice promoted by the Florentine artists Leonardo da Vinci and Piero di Cosimo and the French philosopher Michel de Montaigne. As America entered the Age of Enlightenment, Benjamin Franklin used science and rationalism to champion vegetarianism in the new republic.

In the early 1800s, religion once again resumed a central place in vegetarianism. In 1847, the Vegetarian Society was established in England with the support of the Bible

## DO VEGETARIANS LIVE LONGER?

There is no evidence to show that avoiding the consumption of animal products leads to increased longevity. Most vegans and vegetarians are thinner than omnivores, but going meat-free also leads to anemia—a result of iron and vitamin $B_{12}$ deficiencies.

Church Christians and the temperance movement. The first Vegan Society splintered off and was founded by a non-dairy faction in 1944. Both groups are still very influential in the United Kingdom and across modern Europe. In the United States, the growth of the Adventist Church and their emphasis on healthy living kept vegetarianism alive in the early 20th century. Today, about one-third of Seventh-Day Adventists are vegetarian. The rise of animal rights groups like People for the Ethical Treatment of Animals (PETA) fostered the growth of vegetarianism during the 1980s, injecting the movement with political and social advocacy.

## LGBTQV

The vibrant fusion of social justice, politics, and nutrition of modern vegetarianism has fundamentally altered its values. Vegetarian and vegan are now more than just diets; they are core identities. In a 2017 Cornell University study, Anthony Burrow and coauthor Daniel Rosenfeld describe this phenomenon as the *unified model of vegetarian identity*.[3] Their model helps clarify the broad spectrum of personalities and motivations that make up vegetarians. They describe 10 quantifiable dimensions that compose a vegetarian's identity. Just as with race, religion, or sexual orientation, it is important to consider social context.

The first three dimensions, historical embeddedness, timing, and duration, provide a sense of how society impacts behavior. For example, the longer you live in a commune with a family of vegans, the more you might be motivated to drop (and keep) meat from your diet. This helps explain why many people who bail after starting vegetarian diets live with people who eat meat. The next four dimensions—motivation, regard, salience, and centrality—describe how people perceive themselves. Are they motivated to maintain a vegetarian diet for health or ethical reasons? Do they hate people who eat meat? Do they view themselves as a vegetarian, and is it a focus of their life? The last three dimensions of the unified model are label, dietary pattern, and strictness. These complex behavioral aspects appear outwardly contradictory since vegetarians differ in their diet, but they make sense when viewed as personality traits. Conflict defines vegetarian life. Whether it is part of what motivates people to become vegetarian or is the result of the stresses of maintaining a selective diet, anxiety, depression, and eating disorders are much more common among vegetarians.[4, 5, 6]

Using the unified model, Burrow and Rosenfeld found that many self-identified vegetarians eat some meat. Only 21 percent of those vegetarians who ate meat were motivated by animal rights concerns, compared to 71 percent who never ate meat. While many people who try vegetarianism are drawn by its possible health benefits, those who stick to it are motivated by religious, political, or social reasons. For good or bad, vegetarianism has become a label, and this makes it more challenging to tease out its true health benefits and dangers. As Ellen DeGeneres has said, "I'm a lesbian, an Aquarius, and a vegetarian." Who eats fish. Sorry, Dory.

## YOU ARE WHAT YOU EAT

Once you peel away the politically charged atmosphere of planet vegan, there are health issues of real substance. Most studies of vegetarians have found that compared to meat eaters, their diets contain more fiber, magnesium, folic acid, vitamin C, vitamin E, phytochemicals, and iron (more on this later).[7] Good. The more we examine the effects of the bacteria in our guts, the more we realize the profound effects that diet has in the population mix. New evidence has been found that when the gut is exposed to diets low in fiber, the protective colonic mucus barrier is damaged and the colon becomes more susceptible to inflammation and infection.[8] Vegetarians also consume fewer calories, less saturated fat, and half the sodium that omnivores do.[9, 10] Very good. Not surprisingly, vegetarians and vegans have lower risks of obesity, type 2 diabetes, cardiovascular disease, and some cancers than their meat-eating counterparts.[11] In one study, type 2 diabetics responded much better to a calorie-restricted vegetarian diet than a standard calorie-restricted, omnivorous anti-diabetic diet.[12]

If you adopt a vegetarian diet thinking that it will help you live longer, you will probably be disappointed. Even though Seventh-Day Adventists live 10 years longer than most Americans, their survival advantage might be the result of factors other than just diet. A population-based Harvard University study revealed that SDA vegetarians had only a little less heart disease than meat eaters and did not live any longer.[13] Another population-based study from the University of Sydney of 267,180 men and women found no difference in mortality rates between those following vegetarian or non-vegetarian diets.[14] Why don't vegetarians live longer? It could be because some vegans eat better than others. A 2017 review of 209,298 men and women in the Nurses' Health Study and Health Professionals' Follow-Up Study revealed that a vegetarian diet heavy in sweet fruits, drinks, French fries, and refined grains has been linked to higher risk of heart disease compared to a healthier plant-based diet that included whole grains, vegetables, nuts, oils, and coffee/tea.[15]

Humans evolved as omnivores; a diet without animal products does not meet all our nutritional needs. Vegetarians get less vitamin $B_{12}$, vitamin D, zinc, and omega-3 fatty acids.[16] Vitamin $B_{12}$, also called cobalamin, is important for normal neurologic function, red blood cell production, DNA maintenance, and metabolism of amino acids and fatty acids. It is particularly important for pregnant women and children. Vitamin $B_{12}$ can be synthesized only by single-celled bacteria or archaea. Since we get most of our $B_{12}$ from dairy products, it is particularly lacking in strict vegan diets. Adults need about 2.4 micrograms daily since we can't store it and low blood levels of vitamin $B_{12}$ can cause cognitive and neurologic disorders. Low $B_{12}$ can also lead to high levels of homocysteine—a condition that can trigger a stroke or heart attack. Just for the record, vitamin $B_{12}$ deficiency and hyperhomocysteinemia are found in most vegans.[17]

Non-lacto vegetarians take in 75 percent less dietary vitamin D than omnivores. Without extensive exposure to direct sunlight to stimulate natural vitamin D, they quickly develop low blood levels of 25-hydroxyvitamin D and parathyroid hormone. When you combine this with the typically low calcium intake of most vegans, bone and muscle metabolism can be disrupted. Why not just take a supplement? Vegans skip the usual vitamin $D_3$ supplements since they are produced from animal products. Calcium can also be blocked by vegetarian diets high in oxalate. Even the micronutrient zinc is lower in vegetarians than meat-eaters due to high phytate activity. Zinc is a key player in the cellular cytotoxic arm of immunologic defense.

Creatine, which functions as a metabolic energy reserve, is usually found in meat and fish. In vegetarians, creatinine levels in muscle and other tissues are usually low. Creatine supplementation makes sense for vegetarians since it can improve memory and muscular function.[18, 19]

Most vegan and vegetarian diets lack long-chain omega-3 fatty acids. These guys are important for your cardiac and neurologic function. Don't eat eggs or fish? Then you must roll your own by inefficiently retro-engineering the stuff from vegetable oils containing alpha-linoleic acid or algae-based fatty acid supplements. As we have seen, epigenetic changes in the DNA of generational vegetarians allow them to process fatty acids quickly, but exact the heavy cost of chronic inflammation and elevated cancer risk.

There is one thing that vegetarians do get in excess in their diets—pesticides. A Harvard study tracked fruit and vegetable intake with pesticide residues and correlated it with semen quality in men.[20] Pesticides can decimate semen, and occupational exposure can severely hamper fertility.[21] Because these biocides penetrate and are absorbed into many fruits and vegetables, they cannot simply be rinsed or washed off. The USDA Pesticide Data Program regularly measures common non-organically farmed fruits and vegetables to determine exposure risk.[22] By combining this database, survey responses, and direct sperm testing, the study concluded that men with the highest exposure to contaminated fruits and vegetables had 49 percent lower sperm counts and 32 percent lower quality sperm. The USDA dirty dozen in 2017 includes, in order of badness: strawberries, spinach, nectarines, apples, peaches, celery (a former #1), grapes, pears, cherries, tomatoes, sweet bell peppers, and potatoes.[23] The least contaminated? Corn, avocados, pineapples, cabbage, onions, sweet peas, papaya, asparagus, mangoes, eggplant, melon, and kiwifruit. The message, ladies and gentlemen? Quit complaining and pay the extra dough for the organic produce. Your body will thank you for it.

Long-term, generational vegetarianism may pose its own unique risks. In areas of the world where it has been well-established for millennia, gastric and colorectal cancers occur 40 percent more frequently in people who don't eat meat. A Cornell University study has found a possible reason why.[24] They compared the genomes of hundreds of people from a population that is traditionally vegetarian in Pune, India, with a meat-eating group from Kansas.

The study revealed striking genetic differences triggered by generations of dietary divergence. The vegetarians had developed a unique mutation in a gene called FADS2 to help rapidly absorb and synthesize long-chain polyunsaturated fatty acids from plant-based diets. When exposed to vegetable oils, this mutation rapidly converts them into arachidonic acid. This is good if you are short on omega-3, but bad in the long run since it can cause chronic inflammation and cancer. Luckily for vegans, they get a heavy dose of Bowman-Birk factors in their diets that inhibit the pro-inflammatory and cancer-inductive effects of chymotrypsin in the digestive system.[25]

## THE IRON CURTAIN

Life as a vegetarian is full of paradox. It's not just the struggle they face embedded in a society that eats meat; it extends to the nutritional challenges imposed by their diet. Why do vegetarians, who consume more iron than meat-eaters, consistently have lower blood iron levels and higher rates of anemia? It comes down to bioavailability. Our bodies can't process the iron in plant proteins the way it can process animal-based heme iron. We need iron to make hemoglobin for oxygen transport in our red blood cells and for ATP energy production. Low iron causes weakness and fatigue.

A study from India, a country where anemia is common, found that female vegetarians had a 100 percent rate of anemia compared to 52 percent of female non-vegetarians. Young female vegetarians are at very high risk for iron deficiency.[26] A German study of young female vegans found that 42 percent had severe iron deficiency despite consuming more than the recommended daily dietary amount.[27] In the United States, a study of female college students found that while two-thirds of both vegetarians and non-vegetarians failed to take in the recommended daily amount of iron, the vegetarians had a 20 percent lower serum iron level and lower blood cell counts.[28]

## FOOD PHYTE

There are active chemicals in plants, called phytates, that can affect human metabolism in good and bad ways. They are produced by plants to battle pathogens and other invaders. Some are very chemically stable and could be rebadged for human use. Hundreds of phytochemicals break down into eight general classes: carotenoids, polyphenols, isoflavones, isothiocyanates, monoterpenes, capsaicins, alliums, and sterols.

On the good side, some, such as the vitamin A–like carotenoids, are antioxidants and may protect against cancer and retinal damage from ultraviolet radiation. Others, like the polyphenol flavonoid pterostilbene, may help protect against age-related neurologic and cognitive collapse. Coffee, tea, and, to a lesser extent, wine are loaded up with polyphenols that have significant anti-inflammatory effects.[29] When isolated, resveratrol, another polyphenol flavonoid, has antimicrobial effects and can improve SIRT1 levels. It was initially thought to have anti-aging effects, but clinical trials failed to demonstrate any lasting health benefits. Just stick to the wine. Curcumin is another particularly interesting phytochemical with potent antiviral and immunologic activity. Studies have shown curcumin, found primarily in the turmeric plant, to be very effective in killing human norovirus, and it has even shown promise as a potential tumor-killing cancer agent.[30, 31]

Some phytochemicals are not quite as friendly and can block absorption of plant iron, while others chelate zinc. The isoflavone phytoestrogen is found in soy and can ease perimenopausal symptoms. Or kill sperm.[32] How's that for a coin flip? Some phytochemicals can do more than hurt your sperm; they can kill you. Ptaquiloside is extremely toxic and can be found in bracken ferns, a plant commonly consumed in the Far East.[33] Ptaquiloside, either ingested directly or spread through spores of the bracken fern, directly attacks DNA and causes a variety of cancers. Aristolochic acids are found in wild ginger (don't worry; that is not the same ginger you cook with), which is peddled on the Web as a medicinal herb but can cause lethal urinary tract cancer. Safrole, another nasty phytate, found in sassafras oil, is also an enthusiastic carcinogen. It's so toxic that the FDA has banned it, and they hardly ever ban anything. It is still used in pesticides and is an active ingredient in the recreational drug ecstasy. Nice. Real nice. Speaking of crazy, there is even a phytochemical called swainsonine that is produced by a plant called locoweed, a hallucinogen that livestock find addicting.

One group of proteins related to phytochemicals that are getting some seriously bad press these days are lectins. Also called phytohemagglutinins, lectins bind to carbohydrates and are present throughout nature. They are used by plants *and* animals as the immune system's first line of self-defense. Our bodies use lectins to gum up attacking micro-organisms. We also use lectins to help control cellular movement and adherence.[34] Calcium-dependent c-lectins are also important in how we make bone and heal fractures.[35, 36] Plant seeds are covered with the stuff, probably to help them survive long enough to germinate. Most lectins in nature are tame and have little measurable effect. Maybe you'll get some intestinal inflammation if you eat a lot of uncooked beans. Still, it's hard to justify their demonization as the new gluten by health care advocate Steven Gundry in his book *The Plant Paradox.*[37, 38] Tomatoes are not chemical warfare. They're just tomatoes. Quit messing with my pizza and salad.

If you want real chemical warfare, you don't need nature. Just leave a scientist in a laboratory long enough with something innocuous, and they'll eventually figure out a way to weaponize it. Ricin is a concentrated lectin poison manufactured from castor beans.[39] It is some nasty business and in high enough doses can pierce cellular membranes, causing a cascade of ribosomal RNA damage that gradually shuts down your ability to make proteins. Luckily, most scientists use their powers for good, and we'll eventually utilize ricin's potent cytocidal tools to kill cancers and develop a vaccine to protect us from the odd Bulgarian umbrella poke.

∞

Well, there you have it. Will you live healthier if you cut out animal products? Probably. Will you live longer? Sorry, not happening. The good news is that you don't need to be strictly vegetarian to get many of the healthy advantages it promises. If you do go total vegan, make sure that you get some sunshine, stick to the organics, and maybe take a few supplements. And don't give away your steak knives.

# FIVE FUN FACTS
# ABOUT VEGETARIANS

## THEY CAME FOR THE DIET AND
## STAYED FOR THE LIFESTYLE

### THEY ARE THINNER

Vegetarians tend to be
leaner than omnivores and
have less obesity.

### THEY DON'T LIVE LONGER

There is no evidence that
being a vegetarian or vegan
increases your longevity.

### SOME EAT MEAT

Many vegetarians eat fish,
and some eat red meat
occasionally.

### MANY HAVE ANEMIA

Because humans cannot
absorb plant-based iron well,
they carry a high risk of anemia.

### MOST DON'T STICK TO THE DIET

More than 80% of people who
try a meatless diet give it up
after a few months.

**VEGETARIANS KNOW MORE THAN WE DO.**

# 9

# SUPPLEMENT CITY

"Man prefers to believe what he prefers to be true."

—FRANCIS BACON, *NOVUM ORGANUM*, 1620

**LIFE IS DEMANDING. NO** matter how hard you exercise or how well you eat, you still might need a little extra boost to get the most out of your body and mind. The biggest problem in sorting out the world of supplements is just deciding what they are. I believe that the best way to think about supplements is that they fill the gaps and unmet needs in your diet. Great diet, small holes; cruddy diet, big ones. Some supplements have old and familiar names, such as coffee and tea. Some, new and exotic—nicotinamide riboside, nicotinamide mononucleotide, and pterostilbene. Still others sound like a nutritional alphabet soup (A, B, C, D, E, K, Ca, Co, Fe, Mg, etc.). The blend that will fit you best will vary depending on your diet, age, and activity level, but the same general principles hold. You can get most from a healthy diet. Your metabolism struggles to balance the battle between energy and error in an environment that provides only finite natural resources. Supplements could be the ace in the hole to tip the game in your favor. Don't worry, it's okay to fool Mother Nature.

## JAVA JUNKIES

The most familiar supplement may still be the best: good ol' joe. Coffee, a drink brewed from the roasted beans of the coffea plant, originated in Africa and has been consumed since the 15th century. We love coffee. People around the world drink 2.25 billion cups of coffee every day. Every single day. Damn, no wonder Starbucks is killing it. Coffee contains many potent bioactive phytochemicals including polyphenols (396 milligrams per cup) like catechins and theaflavins, as well as chlorogenic acid (100 milligrams per cup). It is the major antioxidant in the US diet, which may explain its strong anti-inflammatory effects.[1] Science has studied coffee consumption closely, and strong data supports a modest ability to lower the risks of type 2 diabetes, cancer, Parkinson's, and heart disease.[2, 3, 4]

Despite years of supportive data demonstrating the general health benefits of coffee, its effects on mortality risk have only recently been evaluated. Several large, prospective studies have now found that coffee not only keeps you healthier, it can keep you alive longer. Large, long-term, prospective studies of multi-ethnic populations across the United States and Europe have shown that moderate coffee consumption lowers your risk of dying from a host of illnesses, including cardiovascular disease.[5, 6, 7] The largest-ever long-term study of the potential health effects of coffee was completed at Harvard University in 2015 and concluded that drinking 1 to 4 cups of coffee (caffeinated or decaffeinated) lowered your risks of mortality.[8] This study, like many others, also found that heavy coffee drinking (5+ cups per day) did not do much for you—except maybe keep you within sprinting distance of a toilet.

There are many possible biological reasons why coffee can cut your all-cause mortality rate up to 15 percent. The chlorogenic acid in coffee can cut the risk of type 2 diabetes by reducing inflammation and insulin resistance. It also ties up glucose 6-phosphate translocase enzymes to slow down sugar absorption through the intestinal membrane.[9] It might slow down diabetes by increasing plasma carotenoid levels to limit glucose output by the liver.[10] Even though the life-prolonging effects of coffee are not dependent on the amount of caffeine, it may have some benefits of its own. Caffeinated coffee is a psychoactive substance. A typical cup of coffee can have between 65 milligrams and 115 milligrams of caffeine. The decaffeination process does not remove all caffeine. Because of this, even decaf coffee contains between 9 and 14 milligrams of caffeine per cup.[11] Caffeine works by enhancing dopamine transmission in the brain as it blocks a(2a) adenosine receptors and increases the sensitivity of dopaminergic receptors.[12] This may be why coffee decreases the risk of Parkinson's disease. Caffeine can cause temporary increases in blood pressure through its antagonistic

> **ARE COFFEE AND TEA HEALTHY?**
>
> There is mounting research that suggests coffee and tea are powerful dietary supplements that can decrease your risk of heart disease and cancer. They can also help you live longer and lower the chance of dementia. For maximum effect, skip the cream and sugar.

effects on the adenosine receptors, but no population-based study has yet found any association with strokes or other adverse results. In addition, caffeine may have its own unique ability to suppress the accelerative aging effects of chronic inflammation by suppressing IL-1-beta metabolic activity.[13] Coffee, good. On that note, I am going to grab myself another cup and move on to another one of the world's most popular supplements, tea.

## TEA. EARL GREY. HOT.[14]

Coffee not your bag? Tea, a drink made from steeping leaves of the *Camellia sinensis* shrub, is man's oldest supplement and has been an integral part of civilization since it was first introduced in China in 2737 BC. It was first used as a medicine but came into popular use during the Tang dynasty. Tea made its way to Europe when the Portuguese explorers reached China and began maritime trade in the early 16th century. Over the next 100 years, tea became an expensive commodity in England and throughout Europe. Despite the imposition of tea taxes under Oliver Cromwell, tea with sugar became a fashionable and affordable luxury for the masses. By the late

1700s, tax income from tea sales made up 20 percent of Britain's income.

The British established factories in India to circumvent China's monopoly of the market as struggles over tea shaped the Empire and launched a new nation. In 1773, American colonists protested increasing tea taxes by refusing the forced purchase and taxation of British tea. After Samuel Adams and the Sons of Liberty scuttled 92,000 pounds of East India Company, China-sourced tea during the Boston Tea Party, the tension between the colonies and the Crown rapidly escalated, leading to the start of the American Revolution in 1775.

In England, rising demand for tea and sugar fueled colonial expansion across the Caribbean and Near East, trade wars, and the British Raj in India. While nobody is going to stab you over a cup of oolong (although you should watch your back at The Savoy around 4:00 p.m.), tea is more popular today than it has ever been. Americans consume 3.8 billion gallons of tea every year (that's a paltry 169 million cups a day). Hey, we even invented the tea bag in 1904. Unlike my main man, Jean-Luc, here in the States, more than 80 percent of us drink iced tea, not the hot stuff. Whatever the temperature, tea is infused with antioxidant polyphenol flavonoids that can provide some protection against cellular oxidative stress and chronic inflammation. There is a growing body of evidence that tea can help you live longer. Large population-based studies have shown that green tea can reduce the risk of death from cardiovascular disease, cancer, and all-cause mortality (whatever that is).[15, 16]

Can tea keep you mentally sharper as you age? Maybe. In 2016, results from the long-term population-based Singapore Longitudinal Aging Study found that regular consumption of either green and black tea lowered the risk of dementia.[17] An earlier study found that catechins, one of the potent, bioactive compounds in tea, may be responsible for these neuroprotective effects.[18] The oxidative effects of tea ripple throughout the metabolic system by modifying SIRT-3 signaling and DNA methylations that can change the genetic signature of women.[19, 20] If we knew how awesome tea was, we might not have dumped so much into the harbor.

## PTERO BITES

One of the biggest non-starters in aging research was the resveratrol deba-cle. Resveratrol is a plant polyphenol present in small amounts in red wine. Early work on resveratrol found that it was able to modify SIRT1 metabolism and blunt the negative effects of aging in yeast and animal models.[21, 22, 23, 24] In 2008, GlaxoSmithKline bought Sirtris Pharmaceuticals for $720 million to develop an anti-aging line of drugs based on resveratrol, but struggled to find any usable clinical applications. One reason for this may have been the result of the challenging pharmacokinetics of resveratrol, which is quickly metabolized in the liver, thereby limiting its effective bioavailability.[25] In 2013, a frustrated GSK, intent on cutting its losses, shut down Sirtris, effec-tively closing the chapter on resveratrol.

But wait, it's back. This time not as resveratrol, but as its polyphenol cousin, pterostilbene, found naturally in blueberries. Pterostilbene is an antioxidant with better bioavailability than resveratrol, and it has shown promise in animal models and human safety trials.[26, 27, 28, 29, 30] It is metabo-lized much better than resveratrol and has potential effects in improving metabolism.[31] There still isn't much research to show any definite clinical benefits to taking pterostilbene as a supplement, but it does seem safe at a daily dose of 100 milligrams.

## MUCHO MICRO

Sometimes the littlest things can be the most troubling. There are few crit-ically important items we can't synthesize on our own and need in trace amounts in our diets to stay healthy. Micronutrients like vitamins A, B, C, D, and E, along with the minerals iron, copper, zinc, chromium, cobalt, iodine, manganese, selenium, and molybdenum all have roles to play in our metabolic pipeline. We can get many of these micro players by eating a sen-sible, plant-based diet, but supplementing some of them makes good sense to keep our factory humming. Let's tick the boxes to see who makes the cut:

## VITAMIN A

Vitamin A is a group of unsaturated natural compounds that are important for bone metabolism, the immune system, and vision. They include retinol, retinal, and retinoic acid. Phytochemical carotenoids, like beta-carotene, are considered provitamins and can be converted to small amounts of vitamin A by the body. Dietary retinol is oxidized by the body to retinal, then fused with a protein called opsin to form rhodopsin, a light-absorbing molecule to enable color and low-light vision.[32] Retinal is also used to form retinoic acid, which regulates gene transcription by binding to receptors on the chromatin. Retinoic acid also helps your skin stay healthy by regulating the maturation of skin cells (keratocytes), reducing inflammation, and controlling sebum release. Excess sebum allows bacterial overgrowth and can aggravate acne. Vitamin A also helps keep bone marrow stem cells primed and ready to fight off hematologic cancers.[33]

Vitamin A deficiency is common in many parts of the world, particularly during pregnancy, and this causes subsequent pediatric issues. The World Health Organization (WHO) estimates one-third of all children globally are vitamin A deficient and at risk for blindness and immunocompromise. Vegetarians are susceptible to vitamin A deficiency because of the inefficient bioconversion of carotenoids to vitamin A. Low-fat diets and low zinc levels can also decrease retinol absorption in the intestines. Smoking and alcohol can block retinol and are a major cause of fetal alcohol syndrome birth defects. Should you supplement vitamin A? If you're pregnant, or a vegetarian, or both, then yes—with medical supervision. If not, then skip it. The body does a pretty good job of storing vitamin A in the liver, and vitamin A toxicity is almost as terrible as deficiency. The Recommended Dietary Allowance (RDA) of vitamin A is estimated at 700 micrograms for men and 600 micrograms for women.

## VITAMIN B₁

The B-complex family is a large and diverse crew. They are all water soluble and aren't stored up by the body. Vitamin B₁, aka thiamin, is metabolically essential, since it is phosphorylated to thiamin pyrophosphate (TPP), a coenzyme needed to process carbohydrates and amino acids. Thiamin is widely available in the diet, and we don't keep any extra around for a rainy day. When you have enough thiamin, it binds to sites called riboswitches on the mRNA for the enzymes that make TPP and other derivatives, temporarily shutting further production down. If you're low, production continues until the thiamin tank is empty, and then things get bad in a hurry.

Thiamin, like most B-complex vitamins, is used throughout the body, but when there is a shortage, neurologic signs occur first. Beriberi is the classic example, with rapid and progressive neurologic and cardiovascular collapse. Treatment with thiamin supplementation can be curative within 24 to 48 hours. Do you need to supplement thiamin? Yes. The RDA is 1.2 milligrams for men and 1.1 milligrams for women. If you are pregnant, smoke, or drink a lot of coffee, tea, or alcohol (or all of the above), you probably need more and should go over it with your doctor.

## VITAMIN B$_2$

Every family has a jock. Meet vitamin B$_2$, also called riboflavin. Named for its yellow color (the Latin *flavus*), riboflavin is an antioxidant that helps clear lactic acid produced during anaerobic exercise. It also trolls the mitochondrial membrane as flavin adenine dinucleotide (FAD), helping nicotinamide adenine dinucleotide (NAD) to transport electrons to make ATP. FAD is a popular coenzyme and assists glutathione recycling to control oxidative tissue damage. The RDA is 1.3 milligrams for men and 1 milligram for women. Even though we don't store B$_2$, most people get enough in their diets, so supplementation is not needed.

## VITAMIN B$_3$

Vitamin B$_3$ is the hottest and most glamorous member of the B-complex family. Its most notable form is niacin, and it is metabolized to NAD+ and nicotinamide adenine dinucleotide phosphate (NADP). It's used as both coenzyme and fuel cartridge throughout our metabolic system to produce, store, and release energy. NAD+ levels are under heavy stress, and when the reservoir is depleted, it causes many of the worst effects of aging (see Chapter 3: Ancient

Invaders).[34] The bioavailability of vitamin $B_3$ can vary widely in food, and since we don't store it in our bodies, you need to watch it. The RDA is 16 milligrams for men and 14 milligrams for women.

Research indicates that fueling the NAD+ tanks more directly by using nicotinamide riboside (NR) or nicotinamide mononucleotide (NMN) might help preserve energy levels and improve metabolic efficiency.[35] NR is a trace nutrient in foods, but it can be concentrated for use as a safe oral supplement. By tracking the rise of nicotinic acid adenine dinucleotide (NAAD) in the blood, researchers can indirectly tell when NAD+ is being wiped out. When this technique is used in human and animal trials, NR demonstrates rapid and effective bioavailability in humans, quickly replenishing depleted NAD+ reservoirs.[36] NR increases NAD+ levels in the brain and muscle. It may increase insulin sensitivity and induce mitochondrial biogenesis through its NAD+ effects. In animal studies, NR has shown neuroprotective qualities. This is most likely due to increased pools of brain NAD+ feeding mitochondrial and neural receptor recovery.[37] NASA is looking at another NAD+ precursor as a possible way to protect its voyagers against the metabolic stresses of deep space.

Can NR supplements replace the drain plug and protect your levels of NAD+ from falling as you age? Animal model studies from David Sinclair's lab at Harvard indicate that NAD+ may alter the way enzymes and other proteins interact by binding directly to the DNA in zones called Nudix homology domains (NHDs, although I would have gone with NUGIES).[38] Increasing NAD+/NHD bonds may help sustain the activity of PARP1, an important DNA-repair enzyme that usually fades as we age. This could help keep our DNA healthier and avert catastrophic genetic damage. The jury is still out, but it looks promising. NR supplements appear safe and might be worth taking a flyer on. I would recommend a dose of 500 milligrams a day to start.

## VITAMIN $B_5$

Also called pantothenic acid, vitamin $B_5$ takes its name from the Greek *pantothen,* meaning everywhere. This aptly describes pantothenic acid, which is found in nearly all foods, although it is lost during processing, cooking, and freezing. Its primary task is an important one: move carbon atoms. Think of it as the dump truck of the cell, hauling off carbon for recycling. Most dietary $B_5$ is consumed as acetyl CoA or acyl carrier protein, then converted back into pantothenic acid in the gut before it can be actively absorbed into the bloodstream. Then it is converted back to acetyl CoA for general cellular use. The RDA for adult men and women is 5 milligrams. Deficiency is rare and bioavailability is high, so you don't need a supplement for it.

## VITAMIN $B_6$

Vitamin $B_6$, also known as pyridoxine, is used by the body to catabolize proteins, synthesize red cells, and coordinate immune response. It also works in the neurologic system. The RDA for men is 1.7 milligrams per day; for women, it's 1.5 milligrams per day. Pyridoxine deficiency is rare but can occur in alcoholics and the elderly. Toxicity from overuse of supplements has been reported and can cause numbness and other neurologic disorders. Really no need to supplement this guy.

## VITAMIN $B_7$

Biotin, another name for vitamin $B_7$, is needed in tiny amounts for cellular growth, amino acid (isoleucine and valine) production, transporting carbon dioxide, and fine-tuning blood glucose levels. It is easily metabolized from many different foods, and deficiency is rare. Biotin is also called vitamin H (for the German *hair and haut,* meaning hair and skin), and manufacturers put biotin in a lot of cosmetic and dermatologic products. However, there is no good data showing it is useful in that role. There is an adequate intake amount listed at 30 micrograms a day, and there is no reason to supplement it. There's not even an RDA for it.

## VITAMIN $B_{12}$

Cobalamin, or vitamin $B_{12}$, is a big gun. Every cell uses it to help make DNA, weave myelin to insulate our nerves, and produce hemoglobin for oxygen delivery to tissues. At the core of this most chemically complicated vitamin is the rare element cobalt. Prokaryotic bacteria and their ancient cousins, archaea, are the only living things on Earth that can make vitamin $B_{12}$. It cannot be made by animals, plants, fungi, or humans. Cobalamin deficiency can create irreversible nerve damage and is common among vegetarians and people over 60.

There are two $B_{12}$-dependent enzymes that are knocked offline during $B_{12}$ deficiencies, methylmalonyl-CoA mutase (MCM) and methionine synthase (MetH). MCM breaks amino acids down in the nervous system to feed the TCA cycle, and MetH turns waste homocysteine back into useful methionine. When you run low on $B_{12}$, homocysteine spills into the urine and can be detected. This occurs in pernicious anemia when parietal cells in the stomach are burst by an autoimmune disease and cobalamin cannot be absorbed well. In the days before folic acid–enriched flour, $B_{12}$ loss caused even more profound anemic damage in these cases. The RDA for $B_{12}$ is 2.4 micrograms for men and women. If you're a vegetarian or over 50, you need to supplement $B_{12}$. While most healthy adult non-vegetarians get enough of it from dairy and meat, vitamin $B_{12}$ deficiency can still occur in kids or in people with intestinal or liver problems.

## VITAMIN C

Vitamin C, also called ascorbic acid, does not cure the common cold. I repeat, vitamin C does not cure the common cold. It will not help you live longer, ease your arthritis, or cure cancer (at least not yet). Its discovery did win Albert Szent-Györgyi the 1937 Nobel Prize in medicine. Okay, now that we've got our FDA disclaimers out of the way, we can take a closer look at the apple of Linus Pauling's eye and the reigning royal of the vitamin world—vitamin C.[39]

Vitamin C is used in many metabolic pathways and has strong antioxidant effects. It is important in tendon and bone health because it figures centrally in collagen production.[40] We lost the vitamin C evolutionary lottery and can't make our own like other animals. Lucky for us, it's abundant elsewhere, and it's safe to ingest, with tight intestinal absorption regulation.

It also has a very short half-life, lasting only about 2 hours in the blood before breaking down.

For thousands of years, vitamin C deficiency has been linked to scurvy, a disease of connective tissue characterized by bleeding, poor wound healing, and anemia. Ascorbic acid is a key enzymatic cofactor in the hydroxylation of lysine and proline. Hydroxylysine cross-links and stabilizes the undulating rows of collagen fibers, while hydroxyproline bundles them together in tight triple helices. No C, no helix. This causes bleeding even with normal coagulation profiles, since the small capillary vessels become friable and start springing leaks everywhere.

Low vitamin C slows bone healing after fractures by disrupting bone-producing osteoblasts and collagen formation. It remains unclear whether dietary vitamin C intake has any direct effect on bone mineral density and osteoporosis. Despite the uncertainty, several large studies support the conclusion that daily vitamin C intake may help decrease the incidence of hip fractures in people over 50.

Well-designed prospective studies have shown that ascorbic acid in higher doses of 500 milligrams daily can decrease the risk of complex regional pain syndrome (CRPS) after wrist and lower-leg fractures.[41, 42, 43] CRPS is a bad player, causing severe pain and swelling after many of these devastating injuries, further complicating an already difficult clinical path. How does vitamin C counteract it? No one is sure why, but the antioxidant halo effects of vitamin C may sweep up the free radicals that cause increased vascular permeability and swelling after bone trauma.

The RDA for vitamin C is 90 milligrams for men and 75 milligrams for women. If you smoke, throw on another 35-milligram oxidation stress penalty and hope for the best. Can it help at higher doses? That's controversial, but I take 500 milligrams a day just in case. Thanks, Linus.

## VITAMIN D

Vitamin D is a cruel, high-maintenance mistress. It is a fat-soluble family of vitamins that help our body absorb calcium, phosphate, zinc, and magnesium. The most important and potent version is vitamin $D_3$ (cholecalciferol).[44]

There is also the plant-based vitamin $D_2$ (ergocalciferol). Most food does not contain vitamin D naturally, although you can get some from fish. Like most animals, we can make $D_3$ on our own, but it's the result of a long, twisted road trip (Figure 7). Most of our vitamin D starts as cholesterol in our skin, but we need ultraviolet radiation to bake it up to form $D_3$. Patience, this is a local train, not an express. The next stop is the liver for its first enzymatic hydroxylation. Not ready yet. Then it heads to the kidneys for a second hydroxylation to become an active hormone called calcitriol. After this it finally hits the circulation system to control calcium and phosphate balance. It also figures centrally in bone and muscle maintenance as well as cardiovascular health. Vitamin D also helps chelate IGF-1, the evil twin of

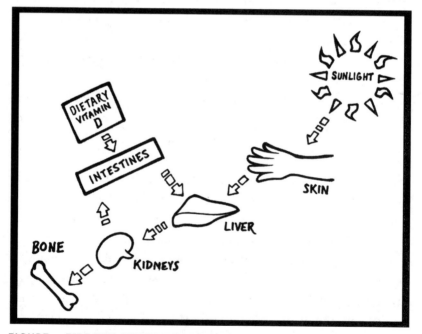

**FIGURE 7: FIRE THE PHOTON TORPEDOES.** The process of making vitamin D starts when ultraviolet light photons catalyze 7-dehydrocholesterol in the skin to become vitamin $D_3$. Next stop is the liver, where $D_3$ is converted to 25-hydroxy $D_3$. Then it's on to the kidneys, where parathyroid hormone helps turn it into 1,25 hydroxy $D_3$, the active form that improves calcium absorption in the intestines and bone mineralization. (*Illustration: Jacob Scheyder*)

human growth hormone and a primary provocateur of cancer.

Even though we can roll our own vitamin D, modern life doesn't make it easy. It is estimated that one billion people worldwide have vitamin D deficiency, many in places with the most sunshine. In the NFL, low vitamin D levels have been associated with increased risk of hamstring muscle tears.[45] Vitamin D deficiency has also been linked to cardiovascular disease and impaired bone mineralization. This can lead to osteoporosis in adults and a crippling bone abnormality in kids called rickets. Rickets appeared in epidemic numbers during the Industrial Revolution as smoke blanketed the skies of Europe, blocking ultraviolet light rays. Other problems from low vitamin D are less evident. Today, we do a great job of policing our smokestacks, but we still don't get enough sunlight to keep our vitamin D levels up. Why? Don't we have a hole in our ozone layer bigger than the continent of North America?[46]

The first problem is that many people spend most of their time indoors, and when they are outdoors, they are covered up. In Saudi Arabia, one of the hottest climates in the world, as many as 80 percent of the population is vitamin D deficient.[47] The second problem is the whole skin cancer thing. Extended exposure to ultraviolet radiation causes skin cancers like basal cell carcinoma, squamous cell cancer, and melanoma.[48, 49] Anybody who has ever put a flashlight against their hands knows how easily light photons penetrate our tissues. Our skin does its best to buffer the risk of ultraviolet damage by deploying the pigment melanin to filter the rays before they get to our DNA. We also have robust antioxidant systems in place to deal with toxic reactive oxygen species. But skin can take only so much sunshine and happiness.

Unfortunately, when it comes to protecting us from cancer, our skin is about as effective as the Maginot Line. Ultraviolet radiation pours through to cause primary breaks in our DNA that overwhelm dwindling numbers of local tumor suppressors. Next thing you know, that mole that used to be so cute is starting to look rough, and a dermatologist is planning to whittle your face. No wonder people are afraid of the sun. Still, you are never going to get enough vitamin D from sunlight if you're inside, covered up, or wearing sunscreen with a lot of SPF. (Just for the record, SPF 45 blocks 98 percent of ultraviolet rays, SPF 100 blocks 99 percent, and glass blocks 100 percent.)

Sunlight still has a stunning impact on our metabolism, even when it's fleeting. Solar exposure for only 10 minutes a day can generate 10,000 IU of vitamin D in a light-skinned person. Think of yourself like one of those cheap solar lawn lights from Home Depot. Just don't get toasted. It still makes sense to use sunblock with an SPF of 45 if you spend a lot of time outdoors. Because people vary so much in diet, solar exposure, and skin pigmentation, the RDA for vitamin D is a very sketchy 600 IU for men and women. That's definitely on the low side.

How do you get enough D? Milk alone probably won't get you across the finish line. Most milk outside the United States is not fortified with vitamin D. Even a glass of vitamin D–fortified milk has only about 50 to 100 IU. That's a lot of cow juice, people. This is a case where you are way better off with a supplement of about 2,000 IU daily of vitamin $D_3$. Working out can also help raise your vitamin D and lower your risk of heart disease and cancer.[50] There are some people who get enough vitamin D but still have low blood levels. Vitamin D requires a special protein to bind to it and carry it through the bloodstream to reach bone, muscle, and other target tissue. It may shock you, but it's called vitamin D–binding protein, and there is a blood test for it. Some people have a genetic shortage of it that can cause all the symptoms of vitamin D deprivation. In these cases, you need even higher amounts of vitamin D supplementation to overdrive the system and deliver it to the target tissues.

## HEAVY METAL

The human body has much more metal in it than you think. It is true that most body metals are present in only small amounts. Iron is used by our red cells in hemoglobin to help carry oxygen from the lungs. Seventy percent of our iron is split between hemoglobin in blood and myoglobin in our muscle. About one-quarter of our iron is stored in ferritin for later use. Men can store about 3 years' worth of iron this way, but women have only a 6-month reserve. We have enough iron in us to make about a 3-inch nail. Then there's zinc, a metal important to our immunologic health. The average 80-kilogram (about 175-pound) male has about 2.5 grams of it—about the same as a modern penny. We have even less copper, about 1.6 grams. Other metals are found in trace amounts, including manganese, molybdenum, cobalt, selenium, and chromium. Iron deficiency can result from bleeding, although a diet chronically low in available iron can also result in anemia.

> **HOW MUCH IRON IS IN THE HUMAN BODY?**
>
> Iron is a critical component of our red blood cells and helps with the oxygen transport system. Most adults have enough iron in their bodies to make a 3-inch nail. Make that a 2½-inch nail if you're a vegetarian.

In contrast, we are built on frames crafted of our most prevalent sheet metal—calcium. Yes, calcium is a metal. Calcium metabolism is complex and extends far beyond bone. The charged ions of calcium help control the permeability of membranes, the contraction of muscles, and even neurotransmitter conduction. Normal bone mineralization requires adequate levels of vitamin D and parathyroid hormone (PTH). Calcium deficiency is common and can cause bone thinning (osteomalacia) and osteoporosis. This is diagnosed with a low-dose, thin-electron beam bone density machine that calculates the T-score. If the bone density T-score is 2.5 standard deviations (SD) or more *below* normal, the diagnosis of osteoporosis is confirmed. If it is less than 2.5 SD below normal, it is osteomalacia. Either way, it means trouble ahead for your bones.[51] Don't think thinning bone is a big deal? Think again. If you break your hip, you have a 21 percent chance of dying within the following 12 months.[52] Those aren't great odds.

Most adults need to supplement their calcium intake, although the calculation of RDA is difficult since we can absorb only about 30 percent of our dietary intake. The RDA for most adults is 800 milligrams. That seems reasonable, but if you are recovering from a fracture or have thinning bones,

126 ∞ PHASE TWO: DIET

you should be taking two to three times this amount. As far as important trace minerals like zinc and copper are concerned, even the most restricted diet will give you enough to get by without formal supplementation.

## SOMETHING FISHY THIS WAY COMES

Fish oil and omega-3 fatty acid supplements such as DHA make up a global multibillion-dollar business built on bad chemistry. You can thank the Danes for this piece of tripe. In 1977, a Danish study of Greenland's Eskimo population claimed that the locals had low blood cholesterol and triglyceride levels despite a diet heavy in animal fat (later data shows they have the same incidence of cardiac disease).[53] The researchers presumed the reason was the presence of omega-3 fatty acids in the fish-heavy Inuit diet. Some trials seemed to back up the belief that omega-3 supplementation from fish and fish oil could protect against cardiac events and even help improve our fattest organ, the brain.[54, 55]

Mounting evidence over the past 2 decades reveals that fish oil supplementation does not lower the risk of cardiovascular or neurologic disease, prevent cancer, improve neural or cognitive performance, or help you live longer.[56, 57, 58] The theoretical argument that omega-3 fatty acids should help metabolism seems solid enough. The brain and neural tissues love these fatty acids since they produce the most energy per kilo of all sources (9 kilocalories per gram for fats versus 4 kilocalories per gram for carbs). They are burned quickly through oxidation in the Krebs cycle, producing ATP and jettisoning wastewater and $CO_2$ efficiently. Fatty acids also make great insulation to speed neural signal transmission and plump up membranes to control permeability. All good stuff.

Since we don't do a great job of converting long-chain fatty acids into the usable short-chain version, we need to get them in out diet. As our modern diet doesn't have much omega-3 (except for fish), it makes sense to get it in supplement form and call it a day. That's a nice idea, but it just doesn't work. There are two reasons for this: oxygen and heat. The same duo that makes omega-3 an awesome fuel also makes them a lousy supplement. As soon as the omega-3 is harvested, it starts reacting with oxygen in the air and breaks down. Since most of these supplements are packed and travel long distances to the consumer, they are also roasted in their bottles by high temperatures during shipping, furthering their dissolution into cholesterol and dangerous saturated fats. A Harvard study of common fish oil supplements found the actual levels of omega-3 fatty acids varied greatly among preparations, with high degrees of saturated fats and oxidation waste products, and was as low as 33 percent.[59] Remember that these are not over-the-counter drugs and their production is not monitored by the FDA.[60]

These supplements may have unintended effects. In 2013, a highly publicized study showed a 43 percent increase in prostate cancer in men taking omega-3 supplements.[61] If your doctor thinks you might benefit from omega-3 supplements, there are higher-quality versions of DHA available by prescription. However, they are so concentrated that they can raise LDL levels if you have trouble metabolizing fats. Verdict: Quit trying to be an organic chemist and get your omega-3 the old-fashioned way. Go eat some damn fish.

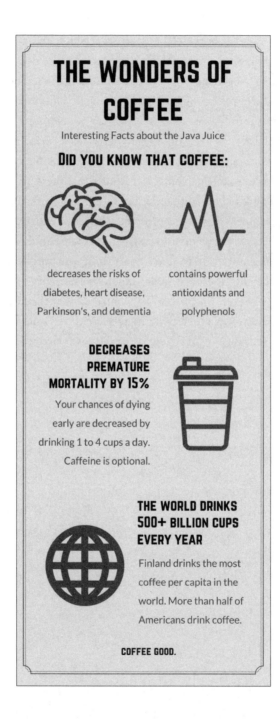

# THE WONDERS OF COFFEE

Interesting Facts about the Java Juice

## DID YOU KNOW THAT COFFEE:

decreases the risks of diabetes, heart disease, Parkinson's, and dementia

contains powerful antioxidants and polyphenols

## DECREASES PREMATURE MORTALITY BY 15%

Your chances of dying early are decreased by drinking 1 to 4 cups a day. Caffeine is optional.

## THE WORLD DRINKS 500+ BILLION CUPS EVERY YEAR

Finland drinks the most coffee per capita in the world. More than half of Americans drink coffee.

COFFEE GOOD.

# PHASE THREE
## EXERCISE AND MIND-BODY

# 10

## HARDER, BETTER, FASTER, YOUNGER

"Eating alone will not keep a man well; he must also take exercise.
For food and exercise...work together to produce health."

—HIPPOCRATES, *ON REGIMEN IN ACUTE DISEASES*, 400 BC

EXERCISE IS MEDICINE. THERE isn't a drug, stem cell, gene editor, supplement, or diet with more widespread, positive effects on health and metabolism than exercise. If the blue zones have taught us anything, it's that if you want to increase your health span and life span, you need to stay active and exercise regularly. The human machine was never meant to be delicately adjusted, carefully polished, finely tuned, and placed behind a velvet rope. It was designed to be driven. Hard and often. We are Land Rovers, not Bentleys. We have always known that exercise contributes to health, but we've never fully understood its true dynamism. Now that we are learning the secrets of the genome and the intricacies of metabolism, science is showing us how exercise can become the mortar of a long and vital life.

The effects of exercise on our body are rapid and profound. Within

**THE ULTIMATE LIFE EXTENSION TOOL**

Regular exercise increases longevity by reversing the effects of aging at the chromosomal level. It improves neural function, metabolic efficiency, mitochondrial production, and NAD+ output. It doesn't improve sex—that one is strictly up to you.

seconds of our starting to exercise, DNA changes occur, protein signals are sent to the brain, mitochondria start pumping out ATP, muscles are calibrated and contracted, bloodflow increases, and alertness spikes. It is on. The effects are not just time limited. The halo of benefits from exercise continues long after the sweating stops. Exercise increases telomere length, mitochondrial genesis, and vital NAD+ resources.[1, 2] It also stimulates autophagy, the body's recycling system to keep your brain functions sharp. It is a pan-metabolic intervention that affects every pathway of aging. Exercise lowers your risk of cardiovascular disease, cancer, type 1 diabetes, cognitive decline, and premature death.[3, 4, 5] It can even help you beat insomnia.[6] The message is clear: If you want to live longer, you are going to have to learn to take the stairs.

There are many kinds of exercise, including aerobic, anaerobic, resistance, and high-intensity interval training. Walking, running, swimming, biking, hiking, lifting, and dancing are all awesome. Yoga, tai chi, and Pilates can calm the mind and strengthen the body. It's dealer's choice. Hell, even curling works (okay, I'm pushing it with that one). All types of physical activity have common benefits and unique advantages that appeal to different people. The cool thing is that the body is so primed for physical activity that even a minute of exertion can have positive metabolic effects.[7]

It's ironic that we are finally realizing the positive molecular, cellular, and metabolic effects of exercise at a time when we are less active than ever before. According to the Centers for Disease Control and Prevention (CDC), more than 80 percent of Americans do not get enough exercise, and half of high school students don't have gym class. We have become a nation of spectators, content to text and selfie our way through life.

## CODE BREAKER

The interface of muscle and metabolism is not just the frontier of aging. It's a battlefield. The simple act of a muscle contraction sparks a system-wide metabolic cascade. Some of these changes are quick and visible, while others are subtle and long lasting. Nerve impulses are fired to the muscles in a specific pattern to promote precise fiber recruitment. When they reach the neuromuscular synapse, acetylcholine flows across the channel to trigger local release of calcium ions. Muscle contraction begins with cross-bridge cycling, a rapid ratcheting and sliding movement of actin and myosin. This is an ATP/$Ca^{++}$-dependent move called a power stroke (Figure 8). The local mitochondria provide NAD+ to produce the ATP needed for this largely anaerobic process. This ends with lactic acid as a waste product that creates the muscle burn of overexertion. Even though glucose is our brain's preferred main course for energy, it loves lactic acid as an appetizer. The brain is responsible for consuming one-third of the lactic acid produced during exercise.[8]

Local reflex arcs can lead to cramping of the muscle, and the muscle can lock up in rigor when calcium stores are exhausted. Training can lead to increased muscle fiber size, but adults cannot generate more individual muscle fibers. Exercise is also one of the only ways to increase your number of mitochondria by boosting mitogenesis and energy production. When muscle fibers are sedentary for long periods of time, they can wither in size. Chronic muscular atrophy, like that seen in people with rotator cuff tears or paralysis, can lead to the irreversible replacement of muscle with fat.

As dramatic as the process of muscular contraction is, the most intriguing thing about exercise is what it does to us at the nuclear level. It hacks our DNA with methylations. Like molecular snow drifting down and layering on the surface of our chromosomes, methyl groups are constantly sticking to our DNA and modifying gene transcription and protein production. We used to think these changes slowly accumulated with disease and were irreversible signs of aging and neglect.[9] Recent breakthroughs in genomic sequencing have instead proven that the methylation marking of our DNA is a rapid and fluid process. It is constantly modifying our genetic signature and protein profile. Diet, environment, and exercise are potent contributors to this genetic roulette.

In 2012, Juleen Zierath and her colleagues at the Karolinska Institute in Sweden found that exercise causes specific DNA methylation changes in muscle and leads to changes in gene expression activated by muscle contraction.[10] They found more than 5,000 methylation modifications in muscle genes in a muscle biopsy sample taken only *20 minutes* after a single max $VO_2$ treadmill run. Another study from the Karolinska Institute in 2014 further outlined post-exercise DNA methylation in humans using more

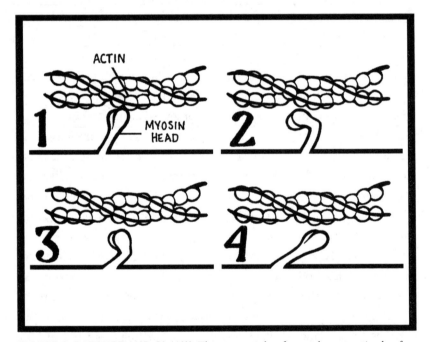

**FIGURE 8: RATCHET AND CLANK.** The power stroke of a muscle contraction has four steps. #1: Myosin sticks to actin at active sites like a grappling hook. #2: ATP powers the myosin head to ratchet backward. ADP and phosphate are kicked out by the enzyme ATPase as myosin slides past actin. #3: New ATP attaches to the myosin, breaking its cross-bridge to actin. This cocks the myosin trigger for the next power stroke on the actin filament. #4: Ca++ binds to the troponin beads on the twisty actin filament, exposing an active site for the next cross-bridge to form. This keeps repeating until you run out of calcium, ATP, or willpower. (*Illustration: Jacob Scheyder*)

sensitive tests.[11] They had 23 men and women exercise only one leg for 3 months, then compared muscle biopsies of the exercised and nonexercised legs. They confirmed that 5,000 tightly organized DNA differences occurred in the exercised leg in enhancer regions of muscle genes that produce enzymes used in cellular respiration, inflammation, insulin regulation, and NAD+ production.

Exercise not only alters the shape and function of our chromosomes, it also changes their length. Yup, I'm back talking telomeres again. At the genetic level, mitosis is a violent process. Cycles of chromosomal flexing, twisting, and kinking occur every time the DNA unzips and replicates. Breaks in the DNA occur frequently and activate a repair response that can lead to cellular senescence and death. It takes a toll on our chromatin. Lariat-shaped telomeres are made up of repetitive base-pair sequences held together by a protein called shelterin. They sit like caps at the ends of the chromosomes to protect against DNA damage. Every nuclear replication causes attritional shortening of the telomeres. When the telomeric sequence finally wears away, the cell has reached its Hayflick limit and dies. But that's not what happens when you exercise.

A study by Tim Spector and his group at King's College in London investigated the chromosomal effects of exercise on 2,401 twins and found that those who exercised more had longer chromosomal telomeres, a marker of longevity.[12] A similar finding was noted in a German study that found middle-aged athletes who trained intensely had longer telomeres than healthy non-athletes of the same age.[13] In a 2017 large-scale survey of 5,823 adults conducted at Brigham Young University, telomeres averaged 145 base pairs *longer* in active adults than sedentary ones—a difference in chromosomal age of about 9 years.[14] When it comes to genetic architecture, exercise makes the cells appear *younger.*

How does exercise pull off this feat of molecular alchemy? Belgian researchers biopsied skeletal muscle tissue from endurance cyclists and discovered elevated levels of nuclear respiratory factor 1 (NRF-1), a protein that attaches to zones in the telomeres that helps them resist damage and to allow telomeres to heal and regenerate.[15] These genes also produce TERRA, a telomeric protective non-coding RNA sequence that is stimulated by exercise as long as there is enough ATP-producing AMP-kinase around to power the reaction.[16] NRF-1 has strong antioxidant effects and may be cranking out TERRA as a shield to protect the telomeres from toxic exercise-induced reactive oxygen species (ROS). NRF-1 also initiates mitochondrial genesis and combines with PGC-1 alpha (a potent metabolic regulator) to promote mitochondrial respiration and energy production. This confirms earlier work that found telomeric damage suppressed production of PGC-1 alpha, leading to widespread mitochondrial and metabolic damage.[17]

In the world of aging, PGC-1 alpha is a rock star. When you have an adequate supply of energy reserves in the form of NAD+, SIRT1 deacetylates PGC-1 alpha, cranking up mitochondrial biogenesis and energy output to support cellular health and longevity.[18] Endurance exercise, fasting, and time-restricted feeding all cause SIRT1 levels to rise, with similar effects on PGC-1 alpha activation and mitochondrial output. The effects of exercise are so powerful that they can even slow the metabolic collapse of test mice with progeria, a fatal premature aging disease.[19] The rich interactions of PGC-1 alpha, SIRT1, and NAD+ drive mitochondrial health and output with a positive feedback loop. All this activity drives mitochondrial fission and fusion. The mitochondrial DNA in the brain divide and more are born with the capacity to produce more ATP to fuel activity and repair.[20] Basically, the mitochondria are running the whole damned show like a swarm of bees.

## GRAY ANATOMY

Regular exercise has been shown to protect neural function, cut down on depression, improve sleep, and decrease the risk of Alzheimer's disease.[21] How does this work? Once again, metabolism is the key. Brain PET scans in middle-aged people who did moderately intense exercise show improved bloodflow and glucose metabolism.[22] This may be a result of the dampening effect exercise has on acetyl CoA levels.[23] In this case, autophagy is more efficient and insulin sensitivity is improved—both key to preventing the buildup of debris in the brain.

Another way exercise propels better brain function is by stimulating gene expression in hippocampal neurons. When PGC1-alpha ramps up after exercise, it floats to the brain, where it drills down to the DNA but doesn't stick to it directly.[24, 25] It finds a local dance partner, an orphan nuclear receptor called estrogen-related receptor alpha (ERRalpha). The pair hook up and dock at the DNA. This dials up the production of a membrane protein called FNDC5 that is released into the bloodstream and is snipped in the liver into smaller, biologically active protein fragments, like irisin. Irisin and other FNDC5 cleavage remnants fan out through the circulation system to burn fat. When they reach the hippocampus, they unleash brain-derived neurotrophic factor (BDNF), a powerful stimulant of neural growth and repair.

Another way exercise starts this BDNF/FNDC5 cascade is through the release of the muscular ketone body beta-hydroxybutyrate. This ketone body acts like an exercise pill, crossing the blood-brain barrier and causing an immediate transmitter release and a spike in BDNF levels in the muscles and brain.[26] The activity of ketone bodies as both neuromuscular and metabolic transmitters may explain why fasting works as a treatment for seizure disorders. It also offers an explanation why exercise can help prevent the development of Alzheimer's disease and other neurocognitive and metabolic disease.

**BRAWN AND BRAIN.** Who knew our brains soaked up lactic acid like a squishy gray and white sponge? At least my nugget has evolved to find a good way to get rid of that awful quad burn I get during my epic streaming beat-down sessions at the hands of Shaun T. Much appreciated. Maybe it's time for doctors to start prescribing exercise rather than simply using medication. Imagine, a gym full of people working out to treat their diabetes and depression. Hey, I don't mind waiting longer to work in at the bench press if we're all living a little better. Too sick to work out? I seriously doubt it. A 2013 review comparing the results of hundreds of clinical studies with a total of 339,274 patients found that those recovering from strokes, heart attacks, and other disabling medical conditions had better mortality rates when treated with exercise instead of drugs.[27]Anthropologists now believe that the metabolic linkage between exercise and brain development may have helped drive and accelerate our ascent to the top of the food chain.[28] This radical new theory is called the adaptive capacity model. It makes a lot of sense when layered onto a unified metabolic theory of development and aging. Our brains evolved to *need* exercise.

A study from Denmark's Aarhus University demonstrates just how powerful the connection between muscle and the brain is.[29] Patients with advanced multiple sclerosis usually develop progressive brain atrophy and have worsening muscle fatigue, weakness, and walking capacity. Traditionally, they have been discouraged from exercising because doctors thought it would worsen the disease. This new study shows that just the opposite occurs. Researchers followed 35 people with advanced multiple sclerosis for 6 months and compared brain MRIs between those who did resistance training and their cohorts. The people who worked out did not have the brain shrinkage seen in those who didn't. Some areas of the brain appeared to regrow after hitting the gym. Why? Who the hell knows, but it just goes to show the multiple benefits of exercise.

There is more evidence of the tight linkage between brain and muscle. When you stress your muscles by lifting heavier weights, your brain responds by firing more motor neurons more quickly to calibrate your muscle contraction.[30] The interesting thing is that you cannot voluntarily contract your muscles past 90 to 93 percent of their maximal contracting ability. It's like you have a rate limiter in your brain set to prevent injury. Practically speaking, high-load exercise is way more efficient at generating strength because of this progressive neural recruitment. Yet we have all heard stories about superhuman acts of strength when people can lift tremendous weight under stress, when that neural rate limiter is turned off. Imagine what you could do if you could nudge that contractile capacity up just a few points.

Now that we've established that you're going to have to work out to stay sharp and live longer, let's look at different ways to get your sweat on. Is cardio still king, or does the throne of exercise belong to the weight room? The real magic happens when you begin combining the best elements of both approaches.

**4 REASONS WHY**

# EXERCISE IS MEDICINE

Despite the clear health benefits of working out, 80% of Americans don't get enough exercise.

**1 IT PREVENTS DISEASE**

Exercise increases NAD+, autophagy, mitogenesis, and PGC-1 alpha. It can also repair chromosomes.

**2 IT HELPS YOU LIVE LONGER**

Exercise decreases your risk of stroke, heart attack, cancer, and dementia.

**3 IT MAKES YOU SMARTER**

Exercise releases BDNF and ketone bodies to stimulate brain growth. The brain uses lactic acid as an energy source.

**4 IT HELPS YOU SLEEP BETTER**

Exercise improves circadian rhythms and melatonin production to help you get some proper rack.

## YOU NEED 60 MINUTES EVERY DAY

get your sweat on

# 11

# THE CATALYST

"Those who think they have no time for bodily exercise will sooner or later have to find time for illness."

**NOW WE'RE GETTING DOWN** to it. Whether I've convinced you that you'll be healthier and live longer sticking to a daily exercise program (which you will), or you're just trying to impress the kids, you're still going to need a plan. What's the best way to go? Running, biking, weight lifting, or CrossFit? It turns out that it doesn't really matter, so long as you stick to it. They all have their own unique advantages. The most important thing is that you enjoy what you're doing. Or at least not hate it. Think of it as your daily dose of life extension. Based on a 2012 Harvard study on the effects of exercise on mortality, for every minute of moderate to vigorous exercise you do, you can gain up to 7 minutes of extended life.[1] Let's put it this way, if I had investments that paid returns like that, I would be kicking back sipping a margarita with Jimmy Buffett right about now, instead of banging out a manuscript between fracture cases.

Exercise can be broadly divided into cardio (endurance) or weight resistance training. However, when you look at it through the lens of metabolism, they share many elements. Most exercise research focuses on endurance training because it's way easier to get a mouse to run on a wheel than pump iron. In fact, we know far less about the effects of strength training at the cellular level than we do about the benefits of aerobic exercise. We don't even understand much about what happens to muscle as it hypertrophies with lifting or atrophies with disuse. One interesting thing we do know is that muscle strength does not change proportionately with its size.[2] Strength training doesn't just refer to picking heavy things up and putting them down; it also includes the broader concept of lifting your own body weight. To be clear, that makes yoga, Pilates, and even tai chi all forms of resistance training. If you can lift your body, you can lift your life.

Can you exercise too much? I'm pretty sure I will never have that problem, but it is a fair question. A 2015 study analyzed 661,137 men and women, including 4,077 people who exercise 10 times higher than national guidelines—that's equal to running 50 miles a week or more. The group of hyper-athletes had the lowest mortality rates and lowest cancer rates of any studied. Their rate of heart disease and cardiac events remained low. So, no, you can't really run or work out too much. No more excuses. Our teeth might dig our graves, but our bodies can dig themselves out.

## RUNNING FOR YOUR LIFE

For the most part, when we're talking about exercise, we're talking aerobic fitness. This isn't just the 1970s headband, leg warmers, and leotard sweating-to-the-oldies kind of aerobics workouts. Walking, running, biking, swimming, and most competitive sports all fall under this broad umbrella. As an orthopedic surgeon, I can tell you that runners are a pain to take care of. If they're not complaining about their feet, then it's their ankles, or their knees, or their hips, or their back. You get the point. Does running cause arthritis? Nobody knows for sure.[3] But there is one more thing I know about runners. They might be high maintenance, but they are generally smart cookies who live a lot longer than the rest of us.

Nearly every study looking at the effects of exercise on mortality has confirmed that running even just a few minutes a day at slow speeds make you 45 percent less likely to die from a heart problem than someone who's just hanging out. [4, 5, 6] A 2014 study from the Cooper Institute in Dallas estimates that for every hour you run, you gain 7 extra hours of life. [7] Walking, cycling, and swimming also lower your mortality rate, but not with the same impact as running. Running helps you live longer because it controls many of the causes of premature death, including cardiovascular disease, high blood pressure, and obesity. All-cause mortality rates are 25 to 40 percent lower in people who run. On average, runners live 3 years longer than non-runners.

Running and other aerobic exercise don't just protect you against heart problems; they might also keep you from developing other awful things like losing your marbles or getting the Big C. [8] A 2016 Danish study examining cancer-ridden mice found that running suppressed tumor growth by 60 percent. [9] Running releases adrenaline, and this mobilizes natural killer cells that hunt tumors. When muscle is stimulated by exercise, it releases a protein called interleukin-6 (IL-6) that guides this pack of wolves to their prey. Why don't we just shoot up cancer patients with IL-6? It didn't work for the mice; they needed regular exercise to keep their natural killer cell populations up for the whole approach to work. Sorry boys, back on the wheel. Endurance exercise also triggers the release of PGC-1 alpha, which is responsible for many of its therapeutic benefits in muscle. [10] PGC-1 alpha is regulated by AMP kinase and is like a master switch for mitochondrial biogenesis.

The changes in natural killer cell distribution and IL-6 levels are not the only biochemical changes that occur with aerobic training. It decreases insulin-like growth factor-1 (IGF-1), a protein that binds to tyrosine kinase and causes widespread metabolic

## CANCER KILLER KICK-STARTER

Exercise improves your body's immune system by stimulating natural killer cell and interleukin-6 production (IL-6). Working out also keeps tumors from taking hold by suppressing insulin-like growth factor-1 (IGF-1) release.

mayhem by disabling normal programmed cell death (also called apopto-sis).[11] This causes tumors to sprout up and grow unchecked. It's great having IGF-1 around when you're a kid because it works with growth hormone to stimulate normal development. When you're an adult, it screws you by giving you diabetes and tumors. Remember the diminutive Ecuadorian villagers with Laron syndrome we discussed in Chapter 7? Born without circulating IGF-1, they are short in stature but don't get diabetes or tumors.

Exercise yields a host of changes at the genetic level, including preservation of telomeric length and suppression of genes that can cause cancer.[12, 13] DNA repair systems work more effectively when you exercise regularly and the production of p53 increases. The p53 protein is a sentinel that identifies damaged cells so that they can be repaired or assassinated before they become cancerous. Irisin, a cleavage remnant of the FNDC5 membrane released during muscular activity, doesn't just cause brain-stimulating BDNF release, it can also kill cancer cells. There's more. Exercise also keeps chronic inflammation at bay and improves cellular immunity. Vitamin D levels also climb with exercise, offering some protection from cancer and heart disease.[14] One thing that exercise does not do is increase testosterone levels significantly. Sure, you may get a little bump after exercise, but it is usually gone after a couple of hours.

## RESISTANCE IS NOT FUTILE

Humans have been lifting heavy things up and putting them down as long as we have had hands. Despite an increase in general fitness interest, strength training is just not popular in the States. Only 22 percent of Americans meet the minimum standard for twice-weekly resistance training recommended by the Centers for Disease Control and Prevention (CDC). It was 30 percent in 2010. It's too bad, because resistance training offers some unique advantages over endurance work alone. Both types of exercise release PGC-1 alpha, which goes around turning on genes like a kid in a room full of light switches. It turns out there are different forms of PGC-1 alpha. In 2015, Finnish researchers discovered that weight training turns on a unique form of PGC-1 alpha not produced during endurance exercise that causes muscle cells to hypertrophy and get bigger.[15] It also promotes the expression of other genes that increase muscular blood vessel growth over time. Increased PGC-1 alpha may be one reason why resistance training is so effective at controlling blood sugar levels in people at risk for diabetes. An Indiana University study demonstrated that after only 3 months of resistance training, 34 percent of people with pre-diabetes had normal blood sugars and kept them normal throughout the 15-month trial period.[16]

Resistance training alone offers many of the same life-preserving benefits of aerobic exercise. Studies now document that strength training lowers the risk of premature death.[17, 18, 19] A long-term study published in 2016 from Penn State found that older adults who did twice-weekly weight lifting had a 41 percent lower chance of dying from cardiac disease and a 19 percent lower risk of dying from cancer than non-weight lifters.[20] People of any age can live longer and healthier by adding strength training to their fitness regimen. Even seniors dealing with challenging cardiovascular and other health issues can safely improve their mobility and vitality by sliding in a few weight-lifting sessions in between bingo nights at the church.[21, 22, 23] Think you're too banged up to exercise? Reconsider that objection. Exercise has been used to improve their shortness of breath and quality of life.

Although exercise in general is not the best way to lose weight, strength training does seem to be a little better than cardio when it comes to fitting into your jeans. A study in 2015 at Harvard University followed 10,500 men for 12 years to compare weight loss in guys who ran versus those who strength trained.[24] The weight lifters showed less weight gain than the runners.

Will strength training make your bones stronger? Sorry, that's just a myth. Once you hit adolescence, you don't build any more bone. The game is to slow down the gradual bone absorption that comes with aging. Gravity and body mass have major effects on bone density; the effects of exercise are minimal.[25] Calcium supplements and drugs like Boniva and Prolia that target cells important to bone metabolism only slow down bone loss.[26] Only parathyroid hormone injections will create new bone. If you do fracture a bone, calcium supplements and vitamin D can be helpful, but skipping them isn't a deal breaker.

The one thing that exercise does do well is build strength—not just in measurable power, but at the cellular level. In 2007, Simon Melov and his colleagues at the Buck Institute for Age Research in California compared the cellular and genetic profile of the skeletal muscle of healthy older men with younger men before and after intense exercise.[27] At the start of the study, the older subjects had muscle strength that was 59 percent lower than the younger men. These older men showed typical changes associated with aging muscle like mitochondrial dysfunction, cellular senescence, and sarcopenia (muscle fiber atrophy). Analysis of their genome found 596 gene differences. After 6 months of weekly resistance training, the weakness gap was sliced to 38 percent and 179 gene differences had reversed. Weight training had effectively made their muscles genetically younger. In 2014, the group at the Buck Institute compared the epigenetic profiles of young and old muscle and found thousands of dramatic changes consistent with the reversal of genetic aging after starting a regular training regimen.[28] Recent clinical research in humans has confirmed that 2 months of resistance training led to genome-wide improvements in DNA methylation and protein transcription patterns.[29, 30] The ability of resistance exercise to build muscle strength, bone density, and genomic stability is so impressive that NASA built a special device (called an Advanced Resistive Exercise Device, or ARED) with vacuum cylinders and inertial flywheels to simulate high-weight/low-repetition weight lifting for the astronauts on the International Space Station (Figure 9).[31]

## IN WOD WE TRUST

In the past few years, high-intensity interval training (HIIT) has emerged as a time-efficient exercise mode that combines elements of endurance and resistance training.[32] Just as with endurance and strength training, HIIT programs vary greatly. Programs like CrossFit, with its workout of the day

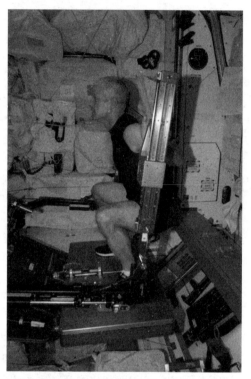

**FIGURE 9: SPACE SQUATS.** You can't even get out of strength training when you are in outer space. NASA astronaut Steve Swanson hits "The Beast" (Advanced Resistive Exercise Device, ARED) aboard the Tranquility node of the International Space Station during flight 39 to knock out some quad sets. So much for weightlessness. (*Photo: courtesy of NASA*)

(WOD), and the video-based P90X are well-known variations on a theme of intense, quick exercises that combine power and speed to maximize results. And the results have been impressive. HIIT programs top standard cardio exercise in improvements in cardiovascular fitness and metabolic indicators.[33, 34] Patients with cardiovascular disease have also benefited from HIIT-style programs.[35, 36]

When it comes to weight loss, HIIT exercise does not offer any particular advantages over other workout regimens.[37, 38, 39] However, an uber cool Mayo Clinic study in 2017 found that HIIT programs improved mitochondrial metabolism and protein production, leading to improved muscle strength in both young and old people.[40] The researchers found all exercise enhanced insulin sensitivity and weight control, but only HIIT reversed many of the age-related changes in the protein profile and production of older subjects. In this study, 3 months of regular HIIT sessions led to hundreds of changes in gene functions, compared to only a few in weight lifters or those who did light exercise. Not too shabby. Although concern about injuries marked the early years of HIIT exercise, it appears to be reasonably safe, with current injury rate estimates of two per 1,000 hours hovering around the same level as endurance and resistance training.[41, 42, 43] HIIT programs are now being trialed in the US armed services and in first responder services.

The verdict? The more you exercise, the better. A sweeping 2015 international study of the effects of daily exercise on longevity found that a little is good and a lot was better.[44] People who worked out minimally had a 20 percent lower risk of premature death than couch potatoes, but those who exercised at least an hour every day had a 39 percent lower risk of early checkout. Beyond an hour a day didn't seem to push the longevity meter any higher. The type of exercise you choose is less critical. Endurance training with an emphasis on cardio is great, but variety is still the spice of life. If you have a couple of hours to kill every day and you dig the comradery of gym rats, then beast it up and pump that iron. My advice is that if you are motivated and don't mind doing a few burpees, HIIT programs are the best combo for busy people who are looking to reboot their genome with the strongest dose of exercise available.[45]

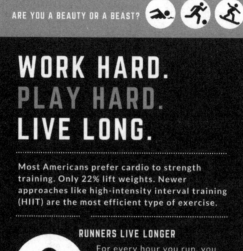

ARE YOU A BEAUTY OR A BEAST?

# WORK HARD.
# PLAY HARD.
# LIVE LONG.

Most Americans prefer cardio to strength training. Only 22% lift weights. Newer approaches like high-intensity interval training (HIIT) are the most efficient type of exercise.

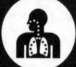

### RUNNERS LIVE LONGER

For every hour you run, you get 7 hours of extended life. Running releases PGC-1 alpha and lowers the risk of heart disease and cancer.

### STRENGTH TRAINING REPAIRS DNA

Lifting weights builds muscle and bone strength. It repairs years of chromosomal damage and lengthens telomeres.

### EXERCISE DOES NOT HELP WEIGHT LOSS

Your metabolic thermostat will not be budged by just working out. The only way you lose weight is to eat less. Period.

## BLEND CARDIO AND WEIGHT
## TRAINING FOR BEST RESULTS

# 12

# THE TAO OF AGING

"The greatest weapon against stress is our ability to choose one thought over another."

—WILLIAM JAMES, 1904

**STRESS IS A PHYSICAL** response to a threat. It marks us. Our DNA reacts and realigns to a new, unique molecular signature that can be measured and tracked. Just as advances in biochemistry and genetic analysis have helped unravel the mysteries of metabolism, they have also provided teasing glimpses at how our mind and body interact. The perception that anxiety, depression, and stress can themselves cause serious physical problems and shorten our lives is well founded.

In the healthy brain, thousands of new granule neurons are produced in the dentate gyrus region of the hippocampus. In this nursery, they are exposed to many stimuli. Exercise releases BDNF in the hippocampus, and animal models have shown that daily exercise can double the rate of neuronal production and growth.[1, 2, 3] Stress and other mental trauma lead to immunologic changes that can decimate these fragile new cells. The resulting DNA profile is so predictable that it is known as the conserved transcriptional response to adversity (CTRA).[4] The sympathetic nervous system starts this cascade by releasing epinephrine and norepinephrine. Proinflammatory genes are ignited during the CTRA, and inflammation sweeps through the system as nuclear factor kappa B (NF-kB) is released. This protein cytokine acts as a first-responder DNA transcription agent and immediately bolts to chromatin. Early in our evolution this was a protective response that gave us a survival advantage. An inflammatory system on high alert could help recover from injuries from predators (or each other) or resist massive microbial attack. Now that our lives are safer and longer, a chronically active inflammatory system works against us and prematurely ages us. Cancer, asthma, arthritis, cardiovascular disease, and depression risks accumulate as the immunologic DNA assault progresses over time. Downregulation of viral defense genes increases as chronic inflammation spools up. The adrenal glands continue to pour out acetylcholine and glucocorticoid onto a nervous system that gradually becomes dulled and desensitized. Glucose metabolism and energy production snarl. The body's autophagic cleanup crews go offline, and your brain cells melt down like a nuclear plant in *The China Syndrome*. Not a pretty picture.

CTRA and chronic depression are usually treated with medication. Treatment with mood stabilizers and serotonin reuptake inhibitors has been disappointing. Psychotherapy is demanding on both doctor and patient, and results have been unreliable. New research indicates that mind-body interventions can work synergistically and safely for a wide range of chronic diseases, including CTRA. For example, meditation combined with running can ease depressive symptoms.[5] In chronically ill patients with limited aerobic capacity, yoga and tai chi offer reasonable ways to achieve similar results.

The more closely we examine the biological effects of mind-body interventions, the more we learn about how closely our cells calibrate and adjust our metabolism to our mental state and vice versa. A 2017 clinical review from the United Kingdom of 18 studies using a variety of mind-body interventions found downregulation of NF-kB targeted genes; this is a tangible sign that CTRA can be reversed through mind-body interventions without medication.[6] Lessons learned from the study of people using the power of their own minds to recover from the stress of chronic disease and mental trauma can help all of us improve our mind-body connection to live longer lives. And maybe be a little happier and kinder to each other in the process. I'd like to buy the world a Coke right now, but it's off my diet plan.

## GHOSTS IN THE SHELL

For being the most advanced species ever to have walked the planet, our minds are surprisingly disconnected from our bodies. Our brains utilize 80 percent of our daily energetic resources, but most of our coordinating body functions proceed at a subconscious level. New research is helping to provide some insight on how the ancient practice of meditation can help us strengthen the integration of mind and body to improve health and fight disease.

A pair of landmark papers from Harvard University in 2008 and 2013 used advance genomic and metabolic analysis to examine the effects of meditation and described a counter-stress, or *relaxation response.*[7, 8, 9] The scientists discovered that subjects who meditated and did yoga once a day for 8 weeks had markedly improved metabolic and genetic profiles. There was evidence of increased telomerase activity, longer telomeric length, better genomic stability, decreased NF-kB gene expression, less proinflammatory protein activity, and heightened mitochondrial ATP synthase production and genomic resiliency. That certainly beats the hell out of fight or flight.

Could meditation elicit a relaxation response even in chronically stressed patients? In 2014, Linda Carlson and her colleagues at the University of Calgary published a study assessing meditation techniques in patients recovering from breast cancer.[10] They found that patients who used mindfulness-based therapy demonstrated signs of improved genetic fitness and prognosis, including longer chromosomal telomeres, improved cytokine production, and healthier immune systems. So, yes, it does work.

**THOUGHTFUL CHANGES**

The mind-body connection is something that we are just beginning to understand. Meditation can decrease genetic damage and improve metabolic output. How much should you do? If you can part with your smartphone for 10 to 15 minutes a day of mindfulness, it will be totally worth it.

Can meditation help you live longer? There aren't any data to directly support it, but improving the mind-body connection seems to affect all seven of the hallmarks of aging (see Chapter 2). The potential power of meditative techniques was clearly shown in a 2012 study of gene expression in two experienced, deep meditators.[11] One subject had 1,668 gene expression changes (1,559 downregulated and 109 up), and the other had 608 changes (338 up and 270 down). Interestingly, they shared 118 gene changes reflecting downregulation of metabolism, stress response, and cell death. How long do those changes last? Given the high epigenetic rate of our chromosomes, probably not very long, but the fact that you can use your mind to hack your own DNA is pretty damn cool.

## JUST BREATHE

The history of yoga is obscure, but it seems to have originated in pre-Vedic India more than 4,000 years ago. Yoga has been freely blended with religion and philosophy over the millennia. There are many different forms of yoga, including the fearsome foursome of hatha yoga, vinyasa/flow yoga, Ashtanga/power yoga, and hot/Bikram yoga. Each discipline has its aficionados. For our purposes, and my sanity, we'll keep it simple and stick to the general term, *yoga*. Today, more than 36 million Americans do some type of yoga, nearly twice as many as in 2012. Yoga moms spend more than $16 billion a year on stretchy pants and other related merchandise.

Most people practice yoga to relieve stress or gain flexibility. The use of yoga to try to measurably improve health and control disease is an old concept, but one that has only recently been investigated with scientific rigor. A

2016 Cochrane Review of 37 randomized controlled studies found that yoga helped weight control, heart rate, blood pressure, LDL cholesterol, triglycerides, and general cardiovascular health.[12, 13, 14] Just as with exercise, yoga has been found to help ease symptoms of loneliness and depression.[15] Maybe that's why people like to do yoga in large groups.

The use of yoga as a clinical tool to help people cope with chronic disease is now being explored. A fascinating 2017 study from the University of Pennsylvania traced the effects of twice-weekly yoga sessions in prostate cancer patients undergoing radiation therapy and compared them to those who didn't do yoga.[16] They noted decreased stress and fatigue in the yoga group and improved urinary and sexual function. That got my attention. Yoga also is gaining traction as a legitimate way to manage chronic lower back pain. This is particularly relevant today since back pain becomes a chronic issue in more than 20 percent of sufferers and opioid abuse is rampant. Regular yoga has now been shown to be as effective as traditional physical therapy for the treatment of chronic lower back pain in multiple controlled studies.[17, 18, 19, 20] Back pain is more common in military veterans than in the general population. A 2017 paper from the Veterans Administration concludes that yoga cut opioid use in this difficult group of patients by 20 percent and led to decreased disability ratings compared to the control group.[21]

Knocking out some reverse warriors could help all of us ease some of the cognitive challenges of aging. A small group of seniors in a pilot study had dramatically improved memory and communication while scoring healthier brain MRIs after a couple of months of doing 1 hour a week of light yoga.[22] The molecular effects of yoga in this study were like previous findings for exercise and meditation. Decreased TNF and other proinflammatory factors were seen, while IL-6 increased.[23] DNA methylation activity after yoga was much lower than seen with exercise or meditation.

There is one thing you need to take seriously if you want to start getting your mantra on with yoga. Try not to hurt yourself. An Australian survey of yoga showed a new injury rate of 10 percent and a reinjury rate of

21 percent, with most injuries affecting the arms and shoulders.[24] The good news is that 74 percent of the pre-yoga pain resolved. Now drop and give me 20 Vinyasas.

## EVERYBODY QIGONG TONIGHT

Tai chi is an ancient Chinese martial art built on gentle, flowing movements and concentration. It is one of more than 3,000 different varieties of traditional Chinese qigong practices. As a martial art, it is measured and cunning, using opposing forces and deception to neutralize and defeat an opponent. Tai chi has also always been associated with longevity, an impression confirmed in a 2013 Chinese study that found it lowered mortality rates by 20 percent, only slightly less than aerobic exercise.[25]

The slow, flowing, repetitive movements of tai chi make it an attractive form of exercise for old or frail people as an alternative to more vigorous pursuits for improved strength, balance, and a decreased risk of falling (by 50 percent).[26, 27] Studies have shown that tai chi is as effective as exercise in improving symptoms of depression, heart and lung disease, and renal function while decreasing chronic inflammation.[28, 29, 30, 31] A randomized trial at Harvard in 2016 that looked at tai chi as a way to control chronic neck pain found it to be just as effective at controlling pain as traditional neck exercises.[32]

Fibromyalgia, a chronic pain syndrome characterized by severe migratory joint and muscle discomfort, affects more than 200 million people worldwide. The etiology of pain is unclear, but neural hypersensitivity is suspected. Many fibromyalgia patients develop insomnia, depression, and worsening cycles of pain. Anti-inflammatories, opioid pain medications, physical therapy, psychotropics, and the rest have all failed to prove reliably effective in management. Tai chi has. A pair of studies assessed regular tai chi sessions to treat chronic fibromyalgia patients and found it improved the quality of life for this difficult problem.[33, 34] Pain decreased, sleep improved, and depressive symptoms were eased with a prescription for tai chi.

While I'm pleased that tai chi can help ease the symptoms of difficult chronic diseases, I remain self-absorbed. Can it help me to live longer? The answers are locked in the DNA. Researchers are now applying genomic metabolic analysis to tai chi to see how it affects our temperamental chromosomes. An intriguing 2009 paper followed people for 1 year after starting twice-weekly tai chi and compared their genetic fitness with a sedentary group.[35] They found that the tai chi subjects had decreased oxidative stress markers and healthier DNA than the control group. A small 2012 study found that people over 45 had 70 percent fewer DNA methylation marks after regular tai chi.[36] Does that mean it will work? While I'm not totally convinced, the evidence is certainly compelling. Seeking social proof? More than a quarter of a billion people practice tai chi or another form of qigong every week. Solid.

## RETURN TO LIFE

In 1912, Joseph Pilates, a former German boxer and gymnast, emigrated to England, where he taught self-defense classes at Scotland Yard. At the beginning of World War I, he was imprisoned in an internment camp because he was a German national. While there, he taught his fellow inmates a series of exercises emphasizing core strength and flexibility that he had developed for his own use to stay fit. Using bedsprings for resistance, his system drew from many other traditions, including Greco-Roman, yoga, and gymnastics. After the war, he returned to Germany and began teaching his system to dancers and other athletes.

Big Joe moved to the Unites States in 1926 and later opened a fitness studio in New York City in the shadow of the New York City Ballet. He published a sequence of books describing 34 exercises, including the infamous pushup. His most popular book, *Return to Life through Contrology,* was published in 1945 and became the basis for the eponymous Pilates exercise system. After finding early support from George Balanchine and other luminaries in the American and international dance community, Pilates grew in popularity. There are now more than 12 million people in the

United States who do Pilates regularly. Pilates is also popular in Brazil, Canada, and Australia.

Although there is less research interest in Pilates than other forms of mind-body intervention, some work has been done. A 2-month program of weekly Pilates sessions has been reliably shown to improve walking speed, flexibility, and balance in seniors.[37, 38] A study of nursing home residents also showed that a steady dose of Pilates helped clear up balance problems and decrease their risk of falling.[39] The application of Pilates as a treatment modality for neuromuscular disorders like multiple sclerosis has been disappointing. A little better flexibility, but not much else.[40]

Where does Pilates fit in for the rest of us? Probably nowhere. Unless you get the rush that Josef Pilates once described as an "internal shower" while pulling on a bunch of springs as you sit in the plow position, my recommendation is to skip it. We already have enough pushups in our lives.

# LIFT YOUR BODY, LIFT YOUR LIFE

## YOGA. TAI CHI. QIGONG.

These disciplines combine mindfulness, balance, strength, and relaxation. One hour a week can improve your flexibility and mental attitude. It might also help you live longer.

### BREATHE

Yoga controls weight and decreases heart disease, blood pressure, arthritis, and depression.

### CONNECT

Put the chi back in tai chi, a classic Chinese martial art. It can help improve strength and energy.

### FLOW

Tai chi and qigong help improve balance. They can decrease the fall risk in older people by 50+%.

### RELAX

Meditation helps improve genomic stability, increase mitochondrial energy output, and decrease inflammation.

### SWEAT

Since you are pushing against body weight, yoga, tai chi, and qigong are considered resistance training.

### HEAL

Tai chi has been shown to decrease the pain of fibromyalgia and chronic back disorders.

### RENEW

Chinese studies suggest tai chi may decrease the risk of premature death by 20%.

# 13

# AGENTS OF CHANGE

"If we have our own why in life, we shall get along with almost any how."

—FRIEDRICH NIETZSCHE, *TWILIGHT OF THE IDOLS*, 1889

THE HUMAN BRAIN IS a marvel. One hundred billion neurons so small that 100,000 could fit in a grain of sand. One billion synapses and 125 trillion switches moving information and commands in milliseconds. Consciousness erupting from connectivity. Deep and primitive subconscious links between the mind and body. Science is only beginning to realize the brain's central importance to health and longevity. Although research in genetics and metabolism is mining the molecular biology of this connection, most of its mechanics and architecture remain mysterious (Figure 10). While the molecular signature of our network remains elusive, the human spirit it produces is a powerful and indomitable force.

Having a sense of purpose and community is clearly one of the most important factors in living a full and satisfying life. The American cultural tradition of separating generations from one another, segregating people as they age, creates loneliness and isolation that takes years off our lives. More

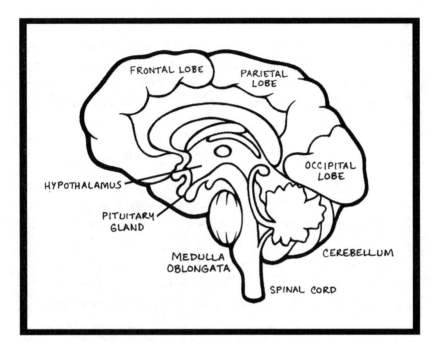

**FIGURE 10: ANATOMY OF THE TOPSIDE BOX.** The architecture of the human brain is complex, elegant, and expensive. It consumes 80 percent of all the energy we produce. The frontal lobe is what makes us who we are; it handles personality, behavior, and learning. The parietal lobe is our window to the world and processes sensory input like taste, touch, and temperature. The hypothalamus is the site of our metabolic thermostat and probably the control center of aging. The pituitary gland is the origin of many critical hormones. The medulla oblongata handles autonomic maintenance functions like respiration, blood pressure, and circulation. The occipital lobe is the site of visual information processing. Its disproportionate size reflects how critical vision is to our evolution. The cerebellum is in charge of balance and coordinating voluntary muscle actions like walking and chewing gum. (*Illustration: Jacob Scheyder*)

importantly, it is a missed opportunity for society to benefit from the wisdom of our most experienced generation. Sense of purpose is such a strong factor in living longer that researchers have created multiple systems to measure and track it.

We are a curious and demanding species. If we withdraw socially as we age, we begin to lose the constant stimulation our brains require to remain sharp and focused. Graceful aging requires generational cohesiveness. Family. Friends. Community. Companionship is not enough. While physical exercise may provide the biologic factors needed to ward off the cognitive decline of aging, our brains need to work out as well. Mental training and problem solving have a surprisingly durable impact on memory.

## PASSION AND PURPOSE

The longer we live, the more we find ourselves challenged to remain relevant. Humans have an innate desire to give and connect socially as we age. Receiving emotional support does not lower your risk of mortality; giving it does.[1] The earlier in life that we define our purpose and the longer we can preserve it, the longer we can live.[2] Think of it like investing in your retirement. A 2009 paper summarizing data from the Rush University Memory and Aging Project and Minority Aging Research Study concluded that people who feel valued and useful live 7.5 years longer than those who don't.[3] A strong sense of purpose and meaning seems to provide better neurologic reserves to deal with stress and adversity. Studies have associated a sense of purpose with lower risks of cardiovascular disease and stroke.[4, 5, 6]

One of the best ways to live longer is to be able to recover quicker after you've been sick or injured. Studies show a 44 percent better chance of recovering from a disabling illness if you believe your life has meaning.[7] A sense of meaning can keep you from getting disabled in the first place. Purposeful lives lead to a lower initial rate of disability and a higher quality of life.[8] Purpose and meaning can help keep you from suffering from neurocognitive diseases like Alzheimer's disease. People who felt their lives were meaningful had improved functional brain MRI scans with less hippocampal gray matter tissue loss, fewer neurofibrillary tangles, and less amyloid plaques than those who did not.[9] Another study examined autopsy results and confirmed that the brains of those who thought their lives had meaning showed fewer of the nasty plaques and atrophic neural tissue that typically mark the aging brain.[10]

**FEEL THE BURN**
The brain loves muscle. It laps up a third of the lactic acid your muscles create during anaerobic contraction.

Finding purpose in your life does not only buy you more planet-time, it can make you wealthier. Oh, now you're paying attention. A 2016 paper that correlated meaningful life with cash found higher incomes and net worth in people who had a strong sense of purpose.[11] Hey, if you're going be living longer, you're going to need some extra dough to afford it. At least here on Nantucket.

How do you find meaning in life amidst all the pain, drama, and distractions that fill our days? Take a lesson from the blue zones. Don't retire. Start a project. Don't move into some depressing retirement home. Stay integrated into your family and community. Tap into your natural spirituality. Join a damn club. Mingle. Canoodle. Gossip. Connect. Be nice to people. Super nice.

If you can't find meaning in your life, at least try to be satisfied. Do one thing every day that makes you happy, and you will live longer. A British team found that folks who enjoyed their lives had a 24 percent better chance of living longer than those who did not.[12] As those great philosophers of the late 20th century, KC and the Sunshine Band, once said, "Do a little dance, make a little love, get down tonight. Get down tonight."[13]

## BRAIN PUMP

The brain requires constant stimulation to maintain and develop new synaptic connections and to keep your cerebellar neural nursery rolling. Can mind games and exercises help? Maybe. Results from the ACTIVE patient study of 2,832 people assessed the impact of BrainHQ exercises on memory in people over 65.[14, 15] Cognitive ability improved 84 percent, and the program cut the risk of dementia by 50 percent. The study also showed that participants kept their cognitive gain for more than a decade following its completion. A Mayo clinic study showed that an earlier version of the

BrainHQ training course led to a 131 percent improvement in listening speed, a 100 percent improvement in visual recognition, and memory improvement that lasted more than a decade.[16]

Sound too good to be true? A growing interest in combining emerging technology with neuroscience has led to the new field of experiential technology (XTech) and neurogaming with the goal of improving human performance.[17] Even though Americans spent $715 million on mental training programs in 2013, it might be a little premature to jump on the brain train just yet. A collection of the best data on cognitive exercise studies in 2013 did not show that they crossed over from the computer screen into real-world improvements.[18] Another study published in late 2016 analyzed 374 cognitive training studies and found little convincing data that they led to any meaningful improvement in memory or other general mental skills.[19] You just get better at playing games.

Most neuroscientists agree for now that challenging your brain intellectually on a regular basis is more effective than throwing away good money on a monthly subscription for brain candy. Save it for a night out with a friend watching a good play and engaging in après-spectacle discussion over a strong cup of coffee. Your brain will thank you.

## WAITING FOR SUPERMAN

There is one mental skill that naturally sharpens as we age. Creativity. Lynn Hasher and her colleagues at the University of Toronto confirmed that as people get older, they become more distractible and less inhibited.[20] I know, you're shocked. The interesting thing is that this leads to higher performance in novel problem solving, a mark of creativity. As attention focus broadens with age, you begin to connect divergent bits of information more easily and with less introspection. A similar combination of disinhibition and distraction is seen in young, creative individuals.[21, 22, 23] One of the blocks to being creative is self-criticism, a function of the brain's prefrontal cortex.[24, 25] As you get older, the surface area of the prefrontal cortex decreases and can thin. This might be the reason for less inhibition and more novel thinking, both hallmarks of creativity. The final component of creativity is a large knowledge reserve. It only makes sense that creativity grows with age. What doesn't make sense is the low priority modern society assigns to the novel ideas of older adults.

Ironically, creativity is highly valued in business and the arts. In the past few years, techniques have been developed to try to boost creativity. One of these approaches is called *flow*. In his 1990 book, *Flow: The Psychology of Optimal Experience*, Hungarian human performance researcher Mihlay Csikszentmihalyi defined flow as a state of mind in which time slows down, decision-making becomes fluid, and mental clarity occurs.[26] The brain relaxes and switches from normal, fast beta wave activity to slow-paced alpha and theta patterns that let thoughts blend easily. Flow is also marked by decreased prefrontal cortex activity. Anandamide (a THC-like compound) and dopamine are released. Thoughts and ideas expand through spreading recognition patterns like ripples in a pond. This aspect of neurologic performance has received a great deal of attention in the military, where it has been induced through transcranial stimulation to help snipers train.[27] The responses in the prefrontal cortex that accompany aging prime the brain for flow states and more time in the zone.

Just as muscles feed the brain through exercise, the brain provides powerful ways to help the body improve mental and athletic performance. The phenomenon of flow is real and holds secrets that can allow anyone of any age to have moments of strength and clarity. After all, what would be the use in living longer if we can't fully enjoy it?

In his bestselling book, *The Rise of Superman*, Steven Kotler describes the habits of extreme athletes and presents eight important psychological ways for anyone to enter a flow state of heightened creativity and productivity:[28]

- Concentration: Focus intently on an immediate task. Visualization and body awareness improve performance. The brain has a difficult time distinguishing between what it is seeing and what it is doing.

Research has proven that even thinking about exercise improves muscle strength. The mirror neuron system in the body helps us model behavior and strengthens our bonds to each other.[29, 30] Rehearsing things in your mind, whether it is a round of golf or the speech at your daughter's wedding, fires up the mirror neuron system, reduces performance anxiety, and boosts results. Meditation can provide clarity and increase self-awareness—both key features of concentration and flow.

- Clear goals: When you're an extreme athlete, your goal is clear—stay alive. For the rest of us, our goals tend to be less defined. Knowing what you want and don't want in life matters. When you can frame the task clearly, flow is easier to reach.
- Feedback: Criticism is unpleasant at any age. If the feedback is immediate and measured, it can help you get in the flow whether it's good or bad. Isolation is the enemy of flow here since it disables communication.
- Uncertainty: Reaching a threshold level of tension is an art form. Too little leads to boredom and too much can cause fear and paralysis.
- Familiarity: Familiarity may breed contempt, but it also ignites creativity. Practice and repetition at any age will help you manage uncertainty, and physical rehearsal ultimately eases flow transition.
- Creativity: There can be no creativity without failure. Whether at work or home, we need permission to fail. The unique bridge between the very young and the very old is a higher tolerance for risk.
- Control: This flow trigger results from calibrating challenge to skill level. The closer they are, the more confident you are. If the ratio of challenge to skill is too low, you'll lose attention. If it is too high, risk skyrockets, fear enters the equation, and performance fades. To give your best effort at any job or task, you should always strive to perform just beyond your challenge/skill comfort zone.
- Recovery: Fatigue is the enemy of creativity and performance. As we get older, we need more time to recover physically and rest mentally

in order to maintain a reservoir of energy. Adequate recovery is needed to handle stress and continue to perform well in all aspects of life. Flow may not help you live any longer, but it could make your life a lot more productive.

Staying physically and mentally fit is the biggest obstacle you will face to living a longer and more fulfilling life. Don't shy away from challenges; use them to push yourself. Exercising your body and stimulating your mind will help you wring the maximum performance (and time) from your beautiful machine. Leverage your natural gift of creativity as you get older and use flow triggers to sharpen your skills. Embrace failure and the gift of renewal it offers. Purpose is the currency of longevity. The real prize here is remaining connected and engaged. After all, for life to be meaningful, it must first be interesting.

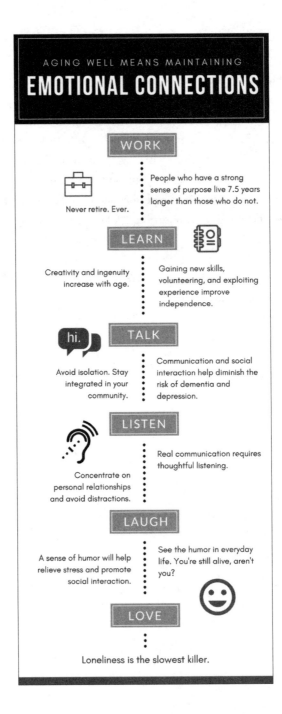

# PHASE FOUR
## MEDS

# 14
# BETTER LIVING THROUGH CHEMISTRY

"It was all about hormones. It described how you should look, your face and eyes and all, if your hormones were in good shape, and I didn't look that way at all. I looked exactly like the guy in the article with lousy hormones. So I started getting worried about my hormones."

—J.D. SALINGER, *THE CATCHER IN THE RYE* (1951)

**OUR IDENTITIES AS MEN** and women are fundamentally characterized by four hormones: testosterone, growth hormone, estrogen, and oxytocin. They drive our behavior, thought processes, development, and relationships. It makes sense that we struggle to maintain balance as the blend of this quartet begins to shift with age. Testosterone, oxytocin, and growth hormone decline as men get older. Estrogen, oxytocin, and growth hormone crash as the fairer sex hits menopause. Since both sexes share all four hormones, changes in this hormonal mixtape present unique problems.

One of the unintended consequences of modern sedentary life is that it is changing this brew. A 2007 study of Massachusetts men found a 1 to 2 percent decline per year in testosterone levels across all age groups during the 15-year study period.[1, 2] Researchers concluded that obesity, alcohol, and smoking contributed to this decline. They theorize that these factors blunt testosterone production and release more binding proteins that together result in diminished free circulating testosterone. When you combine this trend with the natural annual decline in testosterone production in men as they age, you reach an alarming conclusion: Men are becoming, well, less manly.

Women have always been acutely aware of the effects of hormones on their bodies and perceived societal value. They have used various forms of estrogen supplementations for 6 decades as birth control and to ease the symptoms of menopause, a time when estrogen levels usually crash. In the early 1990s, almost 90 percent of women were put on estrogen therapy if they had a history of a hysterectomy. Times have changed. The use of estrogen replacement therapy has now dramatically decreased over concerns of possible associate cancer risks. The latest addition to steroids in the news is human growth hormone (GH). Certainly, when it comes to abuse, human growth hormone is the new champ. From athletes and movie stars to accountants and grandfathers, GH has been treated as if it were the fountain of youth, despite its troubling side effects.

Oxytocin, also known as the love hormone, takes its name from the Greek *tokos*, meaning quick birth. Made in the hypothalamus and released from the back of the pituitary gland, oxytocin is a neuropeptide that has broad physical and mental effects. It helps with muscular contraction (like uterine birth contractions) but may have an important role in controlling aging. Oxytocin also has powerful psychoactive features. It regulates fear, anxiety, mood, empathy, and social bonding. With that kind of résumé, why wouldn't we want to mess around with it?

## MAKING MEN GREAT AGAIN

Testosterone gets a bad rap. It's an anabolic steroid with system-wide impact, including the modulation of muscle development, sexual performance, and judgment. When men feel less vital and have trouble in the sack, the first thing they think is that they have *low T*. When they act aggressively or selfishly, they're accused of testosterone rage. Men are so hormonal, aren't they? The truth is that both men and women have circulating testosterone. In fact, the International Olympic Committee bans women from competing if they consider their testosterone levels to be elevated.[3] As the definitions of masculinity and gender have changed over the past decade, men have begun to look at hormone supplementation. The impact of this on men's health and society should not be underestimated. A 2013 review of testosterone prescription habits during the decade spanning 2001 to 2011 found that most men who were prescribed testosterone supplements already had normal levels of circulating testosterone.[4]

**A LITTLE HORMONE CURIOUS?**

Both men and women have all four of the critical gender/personality hormones: estrogen, testosterone, growth hormone, and oxytocin. Each person's unique blend of the Big Four helps to shape their personality and sexuality. The decreased production of these hormones as we age can have drastic effects on health and longevity.

I know you won't believe this, but the brain rules the testicles and not the other way around. Testosterone production is a convoluted process that starts and ends in our biggest nugget, not the little ones. Men make about 7 milligrams of testosterone daily and women about 12 times less. It is wickedly potent stuff. Most of the testosterone we make is bound to proteins in the circulation system, leaving only about 3 percent free to enter cellular nuclei like sexual crack and do its thing. The other 97 percent is locked away to keep Mr. Hyde under control. About half of our T is trucked around by sex hormone binding globulin (SHBG). When SHBG levels rise, free testosterone levels drop—not cool. The rest of testosterone is transported by albumin, a protein made in the liver. Since the bond between albumin and testosterone is not that strong, we can convert to free testosterone under stress.

When your brain takes in a request for testosterone, the hypothalamus squirts out gonadotropin-releasing hormone (GRH), which barrels over to the anterior pituitary gland as a wake-up call (Figure 11). Its arrival spawns the release of a pair of trigger hormones, follicle-stimulating hormone (FSH) and luteinizing hormone (LH). This pair heads like a freight train down to the testicles on the other side of town. When they hit their mark, the magic begins. Leydig cells start pumping out testosterone like a little sex factory, using circulating cholesterol as the raw material (in women, the ovaries send out a few puffs of Mr. T). That's right, you need cholesterol to make testosterone. If you're a little short on circulating cholesterol, local white cells can cobble together a homegrown version, but it's

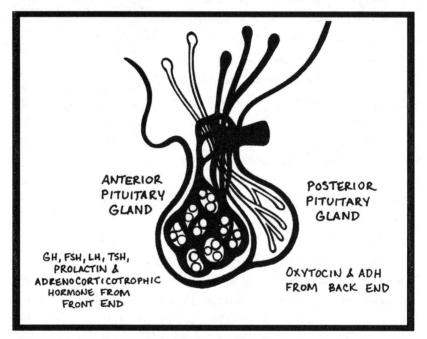

**FIGURE 11: MASTER AND SERVANT.** The pituitary gland, also called the hypophysis or master gland, has an anterior (front) and posterior (back) globe. The front end produces growth hormone (GH), follicle-stimulating hormone (FSH), luteinizing hormone (LH), thyroid-stimulating hormone (TSH), and adrenocorticotrophic hormone (ACTH). The back releases oxytocin and antidiuretic hormone (ADH). The gland has an intricate network of blood vessels that allow extensive biofeedback controls from distant target organs. (*Illustration: Jacob Scheyder*)

a low-quality substitution and can harm your Leydig cells, eventually making them resistant to LH signaling.[5] Omelets, anyone?

After the testosterone exits the production line, it gets shot into the blood and immediately bound up by SHBG and albumin. Free testosterone levels spike, the hypothalamus confirms receipt, and the pituitary gland shuts down LH release. The free testosterone then goes around doing its whole man-thing. Sperm, muscles, attitude—the works. Because the process of making testosterone is complicated, it doesn't take much for the love train to jump the track. Low-fat diets can hurt you by limiting cholesterol, a key ingredient in the production pipeline. Obesity and liver problems can lead to excessive binding proteins that can also lower free testosterone. Even fluoride might be gnawing away at your free T.[6] It doesn't help that as you age, testosterone production typically plummets anyway. Luckily, you do get a little extra testosterone production from the adrenal glands. Hey, every little bit helps.

What can a man do to preserve his treasured testosterone? Avoid low-fat diets. Keep eggs in your life. Eat some fish every week. Exercise. Stay trim. Take vitamin $D_3$ supplements.[7] If you're still worried, go and have your blood tested. A serum testosterone profile isn't the most accurate test in the world, but it will help you get a handle on whether you might have a real shortage problem. If you are low or even borderline on free testosterone, you might be a candidate for androgen replacement therapy.[8, 9] Studies have shown that testosterone therapy can reverse some of the typical signs of male aging, resulting in decreased risks of anemia, fracture, type 2 diabetes, heart attack, and mortality.[10, 11, 12, 13] The results of an ambitious long-term, multicenter study of androgen replacement therapy called the Testosterone Trials, led by Peter Snyder at the University of Pennsylvania, were published in 2016. They found that testosterone supplementation was generally well tolerated and led to improved sexual function, but had no effect on vitality.[14, 15]

Issues of safety persist. Ironically, some research has shown that long-term testosterone replacement treatment gradually loses its efficacy over time and is not as reliable as Viagra or Cialis for raising the flag.[16, 17, 18] Concerns about increased risks of atherosclerosis, testicular atrophy, and prostate cancer have lingered, but testosterone therapy seems generally well tolerated.[19, 20, 21] Whether taken orally or applied as a gel, testosterone treatment does what it's intended to do: get your T up.[22]

Is society ready for the resurgence of testosterone-fueled hyper-men? No way, baby. Citing testosterone's powerful suppressant effect on the brain's center of judgment in the prefrontal cortex, some scientists have concluded that androgen replacement therapy can cause increased aggressiveness, impulsiveness, and unwillingness to collaborate.[23, 24, 25] Judging by those standards, my testosterone levels are probably through the roof.

What's the last call on testosterone? If life has got you down and you're having trouble rising to the occasion, hit the gym, drop a few pounds, and try out a higher-fat diet. Still no joy? Then man up and go see a real doctor. If you get tested and your labs are way off, you might find putting a little extra tiger in the tank could be just what the doctor ordered.

## THE GENE WHISPERER

No hormone is more poorly understood, or more frequently abused, than human growth hormone (GH). Unlike testosterone, GH is a big, complex polypeptide that is produced in the front of the pituitary gland. We used to think that growth hormone receptors were limited to the liver, muscle, and fat tissue, but there is evidence that there are growth hormone receptors in nearly every tissue in the body.[26] Most of our growth hormone is produced between birth and adolescence and then rapidly declines as we age, plateauing when you cross into your 6th decade. The primary role of GH is clear from the name: growth. GH drives the development and maturation of tissue through the action of our old friend, insulin-like growth factor-1 (IGF-1). No GH, no IGF-1, no growth. The Laron syndrome villagers in Ecuador can attest to that. The interest in GH has shifted from its use in people deficient in growth hormone to its metabolic effects and potential use as an athletic performance enhancer and anti-aging treatment.

In 1990, a small study published in the *New England Journal of Medicine* touched off an avalanche of interest in GH as a way to reverse muscle atrophy and restore vitality in aging men.[27] The study found that the use of regular synthetic growth hormone supplements improved lean body mass, decreased fat, and improved skin quality. How does it do that? We know that native GH is produced in the pituitary gland in response to a shift in cAMP or Ca++ levels that causes membrane depolarization.[28] This allows the passage of granules filled with GH to cross out of the cells and hitch a ride on GH-binding proteins that transport it around the body. GH works by physically changing the shape of receptors to unlock and modify genetic expression of metabolic enzymes. These enzymes work in the liver to help break down fat for use as an energy source and ramp up metabolism.[29] IGF-1 works in the liver and muscle to prod mitochondrial activity and energy production.[30] When GH hits adipose tissue, it works to melt it for energy use during rest. Ironically, obesity causes drastic reductions in GH production; it's like your fat is trying to avoid getting liquified. During intense exercise, your brain and muscle have an overwhelming need for glucose, so this effect is blunted despite the push from GH. When it enters the pancreas, GH is soaked up by the beta cells in the islet. This increases insulin production and release. Scientists studying traumatic brain injured patients with low GH have found that supplements improve cognition and memory.[31]

All this stuff sounds good. GH increases lean muscle mass, decreases fat, improves insulin production, and bonus, helps thinking and memory—all things that get screwed up as we age. Where do I sign up? The problem is that from the moment you start producing GH, it's trying to kill you. While GH is going around getting you all virile, IGF-1 is silently and effectively messing with your genes to activate cell proliferation, shut down apoptosis, and give you cancer.[32, 33] In fact, IGF-1 deficiency increases life span by as much as 60 percent because you don't get breast cancer, prostate cancer, malignant melanoma, or other malignancies. It's not just IGF-1. In patients with high levels of GH, like those with acromegaly (think Andre the Giant), cancers of the thyroid, colon, and prostate are common. When you look at it metabolically, GH and IGF-1 cause aging. It's a damn good thing that we make less of it as we get older, because it starts dropping just as our mutation rates and cancer risk begin to increase. One reason vitamin D supplementation is good for you is that it helps IGF-1 binding protein mop up excess IGF-1 in your system.[34]

There are other problems messing with this youth elixir. It's difficult to measure GH levels, since it is released in quick pulses, usually right after exercise or right after you go to sleep, and it doesn't stick around in the blood.[35] You wind up measuring IGF-1 levels as an indirect way to monitor GH production, so you never really know how much you're getting. Then, there are the side effects of GH supplementation. Okay, cancer would be a bad side effect, but there are others. Heart disease, type 2 diabetes, carpal tunnel syndrome, high blood pressure, leg swelling, joint pain, and muscle aching may not kill you, but they can take the fun out of those ripped guns.[36, 37, 38] And about those muscles. They might get a little bigger, but there isn't any convincing research to show any strength, endurance, or sports performance advantage to synthetic GH use. Oh, and unless you have a GH deficiency or an HIV infection, it's against the law to purchase it without a prescription or to use it as a supplement.[39] Jail time could be considered an adverse effect, although it would give you way more time to work out.

All those concerns have not dissuaded researchers, athletes, or Hollywood actors from buying synthetic, gray market GH as fast as it can be made. Global sales have continued to climb and reached $1.4 billion in 2016, with the United States accounting for nearly half of that tab. That's a whole lot of people with GH "deficiency." Scientists have not given up trying to find the right combination of GH and other hormones to keep you feeling zippy, and trials are progressing in the United States and Europe.[40, 41] What can you do to keep your own GH up without giving yourself some lethal cancer? At least an hour a day of intense exercise and resistance training can help maximize your natural GH pipeline. Getting a little better rest also helps since GH is released soon after you hit the sack. Watch your weight, because nothing crashes GH levels faster than a gut. Skip all those bogus GH supplements floating around on the Internet, but make sure you do take vitamin $D_3$ daily to lock down circulating IGF-1.

## MOTHER'S LITTLE HELPER

The most widely used hormone supplement in the world is estrogen. It is responsible for the development and maintenance of the female reproductive system as well as secondary sex characteristics. We now realize that estrogen receptors exist in many tissues in the body and in the hypothalamus of the brain. The true effects of estrogen are extensive and include metabolic regulation, cardiovascular protection, bone metabolism, and weight control.[42] It even helps protect women from the flu.[43] Estrogen is primarily released from the ovaries, and levels drop soon after menopause. This creates many problems for women as they age, vastly increasing the risks of severe atherosclerosis, osteoporosis, muscle atrophy, and dementia.[44]

Men also have estrogen receptors in the brain that kick-start gender development by sensing the estrogen produced from the breakdown of testosterone. Estrogen is what feminizes women and masculinizes men.[45] Because estrogen receptors exist in many organs throughout the body, the loss of circulating estrogen creates many of the problems normally associated with aging. The natural aging process of lumbar disc degeneration as the discs lose buoyancy and volume accelerates rapidly after the onset of menopause. The intervertebral discs are composed of a tough outer layer called the annulus fibrosis and filled with the gelatinous core nucleus pulposus. Estrogen receptors within the nucleus pulposus are responsible for maintaining the health and shock-absorbent nature of the disc.[46] As estrogen levels drop, matrix turnover in the disc slows and the nucleus pulposus flattens, leading to degenerative disc disease and spinal stenosis.[47] Research has also indicated that estrogen receptors in the sympathetic system may mediate the hot flashes and sleep disruptions that often accompany menopause.[48] Low-dose estrogen seems to ameliorate these symptoms and many of the more disturbing problems of menopause. So why not supplement every woman after her ovaries run out of steam? Turns out we've been there, done that.

Concerns over the increasing risks of cancer and heart disease in postmenopausal women in the last decade of the 20th century led to one of the largest clinical disease prevention studies in US history, the Women's Health Initiative.[49] Between 1993 and 1998, the NIH enrolled 161,809 ethnically diverse, healthy postmenopausal women across the country between ages 50 and 79 in an ambitious series of clinical trials that included low-fat diets, calcium and vitamin D supplementation, and hormone use. Women who were post-hysterectomy were placed on estrogen-only treatment, while women who still had their uterus were given estrogen plus progestin.

The study cost $625 million and was halted prematurely when it became clear that combined estrogen plus progestin medication *increased* the risk of breast cancer, heart disease, pulmonary embolism, blood clot, gallbladder disease, incontinence, and stroke. In the estrogen-only hormone arm of the study, a higher risk of stroke was seen, and there was a slightly lower risk of breast cancer. Both hormone arms showed a decreased risk of fracture and diabetes. The dietary and supplement portions of the study showed small positive benefits. No overall increase in mortality risk was seen in either hormone-treated group. The study found that the benefits of hormonal therapy for postmenopausal women were outweighed by the risks.

This led to a precipitous drop in hormonal treatment in postmenopausal women as doctors and patients recoiled from the study's highly publicized results. In 2013, a Yale University study reexamined an important subgroup in the original and follow-up Women's Health Initiative studies: posthysterectomy women between the ages of 50 and 59.[50] They found that these younger women had a significant *decrease* in mortality when treated with estrogen alone. The authors estimated that the decline in estrogen treatment of young, post-hysterectomy women caused between 18,601 and 91,610 deaths over the 10 years following the study.

In the haze of all these conflicting results, doctors remain hesitant about prescribing estrogen therapy. Current guidelines remain in flux as the risks and benefits of short-term, long-term, and cyclic hormonal therapy are balanced. What should you do? If you are over 50 and have had a hysterectomy, a few years of estrogen therapy makes complete sense and could be the best life-extension advice this book has for you. Postmenopausal, but still have all your hardware? It's still worth getting your estrogen levels checked and considering low-dose transdermal patch therapy to ease the hot flashes and night sweats. If you've had breast cancer, make sure to find out if it was tested for estrogen receptors. An estrogen-receptor positive result would put you in a hormone no-fly zone.

If you're skittish about estrogen, there are some other options. Bio-identical hormone therapy using estradiol or micronized progesterone has similar risks and benefits as standard hormone therapy. An example of this is a recent animal study that found short-term estradiol reduced blood pressure and renal disease, while long-term use led to renal damage.[51] If you need relief of symptoms, but have had breast cancer, you can dodge hormones altogether. Non-hormone options include selective serotonin reuptake inhibitors, like paroxetine (Paxil), or selective serotonin-norepinephrine reuptake inhibitors, like escitalopram (Lexapro) and venlafaxine (Effexor). Yes, they are antidepressants, but they can ease the hot flashes and disruptive postmenopausal night sweats. And they are antidepressants.

## LOVE IS THE DRUG

Oxytocin may seem like the newest and most huggable guest to arrive at the neuropeptide party, but it might be the oldest. It was first discovered in 1906 by Sir Henry Dale, when he used an extract from the posterior human pituitary gland to make the uterus of a pregnant house cat contract.[52] Hey, I know it sounds gross, but that's how scientists used to roll. Named for the Greek word *tokos* (birth), oxytocin is a psychoactive hormone that is double the size of human growth hormone. For many years, its only functions were believed to be reproductive ones like uterine contractions and breast milk production. I remember when I was a little kid listening in horror to my mother telling her sister on the phone all about how she was given a lot of "pit" (short for Pitocin, the brand name for the synthetic version of oxytocin) to pop out my brother. Nice.

Over the past 40 years, studies have shown that oxytocin has many other functions. It works in the brain and throughout the body to regulate social behaviors like trust, maternal bonding, and mating.[53, 54, 55] Newer research now suggests an even broader, more complex role for oxytocin in enhancing brain and language development.[56] It also works throughout the body to manage both the intellectual and physical response of the body to mental and environmental stress, functioning as a potent anxiolytic and stress-relieving signaler.[57]

Oxytocin functions remotely like an internal wireless network across a variety of organs. It's produced deep within the hypothalamus, the center of your metabolic thermostat, and then stored for release in the posterior pituitary. After release in the brain, oxytocin dials down cortical inhibition to encourage maternal behavior.[58] It calms membrane depolarization and attenuates fast-spiking interneurons in the hippocampus.[59] This could be one way it acts to ease anxiety and fear. Animal research indicates that it also acts on chromosomes directly through histone acetylation to change your epigenetic profile during partner choice.[60] Essentially, this means that falling in love may be partly due to a shift in your DNA. No wonder breakups can be so traumatic. During physical stress or injury, oxytocin levels jump, dumping out two internal opioids to help manage pain—beta-endorphin and L-encephalin.[61]

In the heart, oxytocin triggers release of atrial natriuretic peptide—not to make you fall in love, but to protect cardiac muscle from ischemic damage.[62] In all muscles, oxytocin stimulates stem cells to differentiate and assist during skeletal maintenance and injury repair through the MPK metabolic pathway.[63] Mice born without oxytocin quickly develop premature muscle atrophy and loss of function, a condition usually associated with old age, called sarcopenia. Bone and fat mass are also kept tightly regulated by oxytocin in similar fashion. Oxytocin regulates the balance between osteoblast and adipocyte development from common stem cell lines.[64] More oxytocin, more bone. Less oxytocin, more fat.

**DON'T SHOOT THE MESSENGER**

A Duke University research team has shown that common house dust promotes the growth of fat cells.[65] I want to personally thank those Blue Devils for adding vacuuming to my daily list of chores. Just great.

The more we learn about how important oxytocin is to our mental and physical health, the more interest there is in learning about the relationship between oxytocin and aging. As we age, oxytocin levels gradually fall for unclear reasons. Given its central role in metabolism, tanking oxytocin production may cause signs of aging due to chronic tissue stress, accumulating tissue damage, and ebbing energy reservoirs. Falling oxytocin leads to stem cell exhaustion and osteoporosis, obesity, and sarcopenia. Decreasing brain reserves of oxytocin may also lead to feelings of loneliness, isolation, fear, and mistrust. Poe might have called it *The Pit and the Emotional Pendulum.*

Is an occasional hit of intranasal oxytocin in your future? I would not mess around with the love potion just yet. Stay tuned, since the generally safe profile and broad reach of oxytocin therapy are making it a prime focus of longevity researchers. The real problem is that testing oxytocin levels is an erratic and unreliable business, with current bioassays showing variations of up to 1,000 times.[66] The good news is that exercise, sex, and caffeine all boost natural oxytocin levels.[67] I can feel my chromosomes knotting up already.

# HORMONOPOLY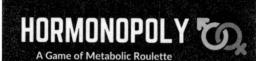
## A Game of Metabolic Roulette

## TESTOSTERONE
The hypothalamus starts the ball rolling by sending **GRH** to the pituitary gland. It releases **FSH** and **LH** that head to the family jewels. Leydig cells there turn **cholesterol** into **testosterone**.

## HUMAN GROWTH HORMONE
**GH** is secreted by the anterior pituitary gland to stimulate growth. It works on metabolism through **IGF-1**. High levels can cause tumors and diabetes.

## ESTROGEN
It provides some protection against atherosclerosis but can promote estrogen receptor-positive breast cancers. Levels drop dramatically after menopause.

## OXYTOCIN
The huggable hormone is released from the posterior pituitary gland. It stimulates uterine contraction during childbirth. Its decline may be the cause of sarcopenia and other metabolic hallmarks of aging.

## REPLACEMENT THERAPY
Postmenopausal women who have had a hysterectomy should consider estrogen replacement. Men with low T might benefit from supplementation.

# 15

# BLINDED BY SCIENCE

"Science and technology revolutionize our lives, but memory, tradition, and myth frame our response. Expelled from individual consciousness by the rush of change, history finds its revenge with habits, values, expectations, dreams."
—ARTHUR M. SCHLESINGER JR., 1986

**THE LAST DECADE HAS** seen a seismic shift in how science views aging. Armed with the knowledge that nearly all the negative effects of aging are connected through metabolism, researchers are looking for medications that might disrupt this web to help us live longer and healthier lives. They're called geroscientists. This broad new field of translational science draws from a broad spectrum of disparate fields including biology, chemistry, physics, and medicine.[1] When scientists view the process of getting older as a disease, new and old medications can be developed, evaluated, and compared rigorously. Research in geroscience is focusing on five broad medical approaches to life and health extension:[2]

- Antioxidants
- Telomerase activators

- Autophagy activators
- Senolytics
- Calorie-restriction mimetics

Most models of aging acknowledge that oxidative stress damage from free radicals causes harm to mitochondrial DNA, resulting in energy losses that affect all body tissues. Drugs that can reduce the levels of oxidative stress or activate oxidative resistance could be extremely valuable in improving cellular health. Although the impact of antioxidant supplements has been disappointing so far, the use of melatonin may hold some promise. Melatonin is a native hormone released in pulses from the pineal gland during sleep. It helps regulate circadian rhythm and SIRT1 activation. The best way to stimulate melatonin naturally is to work out, but it takes some time for it to build up. You need at least an hour to get it rolling.

The tight linkage between telomeric length and chromosomal integrity makes this an attractive area for investigation. Telomerase is a specialized reverse transcriptase that can help the telomeres from wearing away during cellular division. Early research has shown that telomerase activators work effectively to repair defective telomerase enzyme production and lengthen life span by as much as 40 percent in knockout mice, but they cause too much cellular growth in normal mice, leading to cancer. Current research is looking for ways to shortcut tumor genesis from telomerase activation while still gaining DNA protection.

The autophagy system is a complex recycling network used to identify, kill, and reuse damaged cells and proteins. Breakdown of this machinery is one of the primary hallmarks of aging and is a metabolic disaster for the body, leading to the accumulation of toxins and debris. Alzheimer's, Parkinson's, renal disease, and many other devastating disorders of aging result from the loss of autophagy. Several suitors for autophagic induction are now being evaluated, including spermidine, ethanolamine, and beta-guanidinopropionic acid. Rapamycin also helps cellular fitness by improving autophagy.

The two remaining focal points of geroscience—senolytic and calorie-restriction mimetic meds—deserve closer attention as they hurtle toward mainstream use. Up until recently, most senolytics have pulled double duty as chemotherapy drugs. This meant they were good at killing things. Unfortunately, while they could blow up senescent cells, they also did a job on normal platelets. Now a whole new breed of senolytics is coming to biotech start-ups around the globe.

## SPRING CLEANING

Life is hard on our little Lego blocks. Environmental or metabolic stress can damage DNA enough to initiate a cellular shutdown called senescence.[3] These damaged, dying, or precancerous cells must be killed and removed by our immune system to make room for new cells. At any one time as many as 15 percent of our cells are senescent. For half a century, scientists have been working to try to unravel their connection to aging and disease. In 2011, a team at the Mayo Clinic fluorescently tagged these cells and tracked their accumulation in cataracts, arterial plaques, and other aging issue.[4] Now they have been able to use targeted experimental drugs to flip the genetic switch in the DNA of the beat-up cells, heading off their path to cancer and inflammation.[5] Mice loaded with senescent cells show premature aging. When they were treated with genetically targeted manipulation, the senescent cells were killed and signs of aging resolved.

In healthy organisms, senescent cells are constantly being hunted by an assassin protein called p53. New research shows that this guardian of the genome, which was first discovered in 1979, listens in for faint changes in DNA oscillation that signal damage.[6] The stakes are high in this genetic game of cat and mouse. If the senescent cells escape, they elicit an intense inflammatory response that can be lethal. Senescent foam cells in coronary artery plaques can cause massive ischemic damage. When senescent cells are found, the p53 proteins engulf them, and they are eaten by white cells from our immune system.[7] But it seems that senescent cells have a strong sense of self-preservation. Since they can't run, some of these damaged cells trigger FOXO4 proteins to stick to the p53 surface, which helps them evade the immune system's roaming sentinel macrophages. A group of Dutch scientists have engineered a FOXO4-blocking peptide fragment that fills the surface receptor clefts and escorts the p53 protein clear of FOXO4.[8] This allows apoptosis and cellular recycling to continue unfettered.

What happens when our p53 jaegers get banged up and stop minding the shop? Bad things. Very bad things. As many as half of all cancers are associated with mutated p53. While most research has focused on propping up levels of healthy p53, new drugs are being used to fix the damaged p53 so it can get back to work. Most of these have focused on restoring the shape of p53 and their ability to attach to damaged DNA molecules. By adding zinc to the core of floppy p53 proteins, they hold their shape better to allow better adherence to broken DNA.

Senescent macrophages full of lipids lodge in coronary arteries. After they burrow into the plaque wall, these nasty foam cells, swollen with fat, cause an aggressive inflammatory response and cardiac damage.[9] Targeted senolytics have been shown to decrease coronary plaques by 60 percent in animal models. It turns out that a little roto-rooter action might help your joints as well. Senescent cells appear to play a critical role in the progression of osteoarthritis. Early experimental work with a senolytic called UBX0101 showed improvement with arthritic symptoms after joint injection.[10] Senolytic research has expanded into pulmonary and renal disease, with clinical trials in humans on the horizon.[11]

Despite the encouraging early results in animal models, many hurdles remain before senolytics go mainstream. Many are peptides easily broken down by the digestive system. Others cause too much collateral damage to healthy cells. Success can be as problematic as failure. In the heart, one of the real problems will be to ward off clumps of dead, senescent cell plaques breaking free. These cardiac icebergs could block arteries, causing strokes or blood clots. Because senolytics seem to reverse many of the hallmarks of aging, research will continue to examine new models and applications for treatment.[12, 13, 14]

## STAYIN' ALIVE

The excitement and enthusiasm regarding senolytics have eclipsed the first anti-aging drug to be evaluated in an FDA clinical trial—metformin. Also known by its trade name, Glucophage, metformin seems almost nostalgic compared to exotic brews like UBX0101. Its origins lie in an invasive weed,

French lilac, used for hundreds of years as a folk medicine to treat a wide assortment of ailments. More than 80 million Americans now use metformin to treat type 2 diabetes. Researchers discovered an unintended side effect of the drug—patients had far fewer cancers compared to those without diabetes not taking metformin.[15] The cool thing here isn't just that metformin controls diabetes and cuts down on cancer. It's that metformin may realize the real hope of longevity researchers: to improve our health span and life quality as we age.[16]

How does metformin impact aging? This is one metabolic multitasking mega-machine. Its primary effect is to drop insulin levels and control blood glucose levels. This helps prevent high blood sugar from overwhelming cells, forcing them to be more fuel efficient. Less obesity is good because it means less cancer, less heart disease, and less dying. It also suppresses IGF-1, that sneaky cancer promoter and clarion for all things that suck about aging.[17]

Metformin may protect against pancreatic cancer because it blocks transcription of genes that signal mTOR (for more on mTOR, see page 196).[18] This chokes off resources that encourage tumor initiation and unbridled growth. It also works metabolically via AMPK pathway activation to turn on SIRT1, slashes oxidative stress during mitochondrial energy production, and decreases DNA mutation rates.[19, 20, 21] All these pathways lead to less error and more available energy, the keys to longevity and health.

I see you hovering that mouse over that Mexican metformin banner. Keep your shirt on, gringo. The FDA has finally admitted that medications that decrease the negative effects of aging are worthy of study. The Targeting Aging with Metformin (TAME) clinical trial to assess metformin's overall performance as an anti-aging drug is now under way under the direction of Dr. Nir Barzilai at the Albert Einstein College of Medicine in New York City. Let the man do his work, and we'll see if the benefits outweigh the risks.

**LIVES OF A MED**

Metformin, a medication used to treat diabetes, is the first drug to enter a clinical trial with the FDA as a targeted anti-aging treatment. It improves nutrient sensitivity and energy management. It also suppresses IGF-1 and mTOR to dial up longevity, making it a potent calorie-restriction mimetic candidate.

# 5 APPROACHES TO CONTROL
# AGING

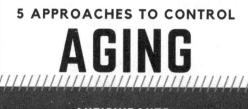

## ANTIOXIDANTS

High-dose antioxidant treatments have not proved rewarding to date. The newest candidate is melatonin, which is produced naturally during exercise & sleep.

## TELOMERASE INHIBITORS

Preserving telomeric length could allow cells to avoid reaching the "Hayflick limit" and survive indefinitely. The problem is that tumor cells already do this, and cancer is a lethal side effect.

## AUTOPHAGY ACTIVATORS

This is a promising area of research since they could also help reduce dementia and Parkinson's. Spermadine and ethanolamine are prime candidates.

## SENOLYTICS

These drugs are the hottest new players in the anti-aging sandbox. Senolytics are designed to clean out dead cells before they can cause inflammation and secondary heart disease.

## CALORIE-RESTRICTION MIMETICS

Metformin is the first FDA anti-aging trial.

# 16
## STRANGER THINGS

"Not a soul was to be seen on shore, only a deserted, petrified world with motionless stone heads gazing at us from their distant ridge . . . The shadows were long, but nothing moved; nothing but the fiery red sun as it descended slowly into the black sea."
—THOR HEYERDAHL, *AKU-AKU*, 1958

**THE STORY OF** *THE Fountain* ends much as it began—on a harsh, isolated island that might hold the key to unlocking the secrets of aging. Easter Island is a tiny spit of land located 2,200 miles off the coast of Chile in the vast emptiness of the southeastern Pacific Ocean. Also known as Rapa Nui, a named derived from its original inhabitants, the windswept, volcanic triangle of land is known for its ancient monolithic statues, the moai, and scattered stone temples, the ahu. The true story of this remote island and its impact on the future of the science of aging and medicine is more bizarre than any fictional tale. Meet rapamycin and the object of its affection and ground zero in the fight for longevity, mTOR.

Aging casts a wide metabolic net. Innovative approaches are evolving to disable its effects in a broad new range of medications and treatments. By throwing a genetic switch and combining it with exercise, scientists are beginning to grow brain tissue once thought to be irrevocably damaged. The perception of pain has an extraordinary effect on metabolism and aging. The targeted suppression of pain sensors may improve our health span. As the story of rapamycin demonstrates, pharmaceutical research has traditionally focused on remote regions of the world to make new medical discoveries. Now scientists are mining trillions of bacteria that populate the microbiome of our bodies in hopes of new compounds in the brave new world of inner space.

## SILENT SENTINELS

Easter Island was first populated by migratory Polynesians around 1100 AD, who called it Aku-Aku. The island initially thrived, and the population swelled to 15,000. A warrior class system rose that built the moai, the giant enigmatic human statues that define the island, and the mysterious stone shrines called ahus. Centuries of deforestation, cannibalism, and internal strife followed that eroded the ecosystem and infrastructure of the island. By the time the island was discovered by Dutch explorers in 1722, the population had contracted to an estimated 3,000 inhabitants (minus the 12 natives the Europeans killed on opening day of their weeklong visit). Subsequent flybys by Spanish and English ships over the next 100 years were met with violence. In 1862, Peruvian pirate ships assisted by the Spanish frigate *Rosa y Carmen* made landfall and abducted more than 1,500 men and women for the slave trade in a raid that lasted several months. This disaster was compounded when some slaves carrying smallpox and tuberculosis were repatriated to the island in 1865. Within a decade, 97 percent of the island's population were dead or had fled the pestilence with the help of missionaries. In 1888, Chile annexed the skeletonized island and limited the few remaining natives to the small settlement of Hanga Roa. The rest of the island was devoted to sheep and horse farming. With no natural ports, the island was virtually isolated for the next century except for sporadic supply ship runs from the Chilean mainland.

# VOYAGE TO THE END OF THE WORLD

Nothing attracts biologists like isolation. So rare in the modern world, isolation allows scientists to track genetics and hereditary patterns in unique ways. The Easter Island of the mid-20th century, surrounded by the imposing barrier of the Pacific Ocean and devoid of even rudimentary communications, seemed the perfect living laboratory to study the effects of environment on man. It first attracted the attention of Dr. Stanley C. Skoryna, an associate professor in gastrointestinal disorders at Montreal's McGill University, in 1961.[1] When he learned that Chile intended to build an airstrip on Easter Island to facilitate trade with Australia, Skoryna began to assemble an expedition to catalogue the island's biology before it became contaminated by off-islanders. He was interested in finding a possible link between ulcers and stomach cancer and combined his efforts with Dr. Georges Nógrady, a bacteriologist from the University of Montreal. Nógrady and his colleagues were interested in studying tetanus, leprosy, tuberculosis, whooping cough, and fungal diseases. This set into motion an unprecedented collaboration that led to the creation of the Medical Expedition to Easter Island (METEI).

At the time, the World Health Organization (WHO) was in the thick of the Human Adaptability Section of their international biological program studying the relationship between man and environment. The WHO kickstarted the project with a $5,000 pilot grant, and METEI was born. Skoryna formed the Easter Island Expedition Society in 1963 and began raising the massive amount of capital needed to fund his adventure. Money and lab equipment flowed into the society from a broad range of sources including McGill University, General Motors, Dupont, and the Canadian government. The Alberta Trailer Company donated 24 palletized trailers as living and working modules. The Canadian Royal Navy provided a 48-foot landing craft and refitted the 8,100-ton repair ship *Cape Scott* with double the fuel capacity and additional storage space for the long trek. As interest grew, the crew expanded to a full complement of 38 that included scientists, support staff, and a *Life* magazine photographer. Tons of fuel, food, and equipment, including diesel generators, x-ray machines, and water recyclers, were procured and loaded. The Canadian Armed Forces took over control of the burgeoning expedition. The METEI journey began as the *Cape Scott* sailed out of Halifax on a crisp November morning in 1964.

She crossed the Panama Canal and arrived at Easter Island 1 month later, on December 13, making anchor in Cook's Bay, near Hanga Roa. Total island drama ensued. When they made landfall, the island was in the midst of political upheaval. No supply ships had been to the island for more than a year, and there were island-wide shortages of food and toiletries. With the help of local Roman Catholic priests, Skoryna distributed 200 parcels of the expedition's food to help feed the islanders. Despite this goodwill, the growing animosity between the Rapanui and Chileans threatened the expedition. After the METEI team set up camp, the *Cape Scott* left for the nearest port of Valparaiso. It was supposed to return an old bulldozer to the mainland, but one of the local teachers hijacked some vital parts. With the bulldozer stranded on the beach, the island's powerful governor, Jorge Portilla, lost his mind, and word of a revolution soon reached Santiago. Human research was suspended.

During this time, Georges Nógrady kept busy. He was looking for tetanus. Typically, tetanus is spread from horses to humans via ground-based spores that enter the bloodstream through small cuts or abrasions. Given the large number of horses, sharp volcanic terrain, and barefooted preference of the Rapanui, tetanus should have been common on Easter Island. Nógrady didn't find any spores testing around the base camp. He then divided the island into 64 parcels and carefully collected soil samples from the center of each section. The samples were catalogued and packed away in a deep medical freezer for transport back to Canada.

A Chilean arctic patrol boat with 40 marines was met with antagonism when it arrived on January 5. After a warning shot dispersed a boisterous crowd on January 8, the "delightful revolution" was amicably quelled, ending with ceremonial leis and a conciliatory round of municipal elections. The research resumed, and the METEI researchers completed their ambitious mission over the ensuing 4 weeks, obtaining histories, swabs, bloodwork, and x-rays from all of the island's inhabitants. The *Cape Scott* returned to Easter Island on February 10, 1965, to pick up the scientists, crew, and samples and set sail for Canada 2 days later, leaving the trailers and heavy equipment behind.[2]

Okay, so I admit it isn't as good a story as the movie *Anaconda*, but it is still *way* better than *Anaconda 2, 3,* or *4*. While we might be missing the blood orchid of eternal life and a really big snake (as well as the incomparable cast of J. Lo, Eric Stoltz, and Ice Cube), we do get a cancer-killing star of our own. Rapamycin.

## DO NOT EAT

When Georges Nógrady returned to Canada, he sent 72 soil samples from Easter Island to a Virginia lab for analysis. Only one was positive for tetanus spores, and he found no evidence of tuberculosis. Satisfied with the answer that tetanus was rare on Rapa Nui, he put the remaining samples into deep frozen storage and returned to his work analyzing the human test data. Skoryna, deeply in debt after the mission, scrambled to pay off his bills from the expedition and lost interest in any follow-up. No papers were published. METEI was over. The real irony is that it took nearly another half-century before researchers finally found the bacterial link between stomach ulcers and cancer that had eluded Skoryna.

In 1972, an accomplished Indian-born Canadian scientist named Suren Sehgal, working for the giant pharmaceutical company Ayerst, somehow got his hands on the old frozen METEI soil samples for analysis. He isolated bacteria called *Streptomyces hygroscopicus* from one sample and found that the little guys secreted a number of unique, bioactive peptides. One of these chemicals, AY-22,989, demonstrated aggressive antifungal properties and potent tumor-killing ability.[3] He named his newly adopted molecular child rapamycin, after the island of its origin. Confident that it could have even broader use as a cancer drug, he sent it to the National Cancer Institute for a tumor-killing assay. The NCI was impressed. Unfortunately, Ayerst, a pharmaceutical company, was not. Under heavy financial burden and steered by new management, Ayerst shut down its Canadian operations and laid off 95 percent of its workforce. Sehgal survived the cut, which means the dude was smart. Even smarter was that when he left the land of the maple leaf, he took the last few frozen vials of his beloved rapamycin with him. That was a good call, since the company had marked it as a "nonviable" drug slated for destruction. When he moved with his family to New Jersey, he had a serious mad scientist moment. He stashed some stolen rapamycin in a plastic bag labeled in black marker, "Do Not Eat," and hid it in the back of his home freezer. Right behind the ice cream.

In 1987, Wyeth Pharmaceuticals gobbled up Ayerst, and it was game on for rapamycin. Hungry for a new pipeline drug, Sehgal dug his rapamycin out of the fridge, and Wyeth resurrected it as sirolimus. The main problem for rapamycin and all its relatives (called rapalogs) is that they don't just kill tumors, they kill everything. The powerful immunosuppressant traits of rapamycin were problematic. Now if you're dying from some crazy tumor, crashing the entire immune system is a risk you don't mind taking. However, if all you're looking for is something new to knock out athlete's foot, it might give you a reason to reconsider. Despite its potentially catastrophic side effects, Sehgal did not abandon his sire.

Chemists have a saying: "Never let a good side effect go to waste." The booming growth of organ transplants in the United States during the 1990s was hampered by lingering problems with host rejection of donor tissue. Stronger immunosuppressants were needed. Sehgal and Wyeth saw an opportunity. In 1999, the FDA approved a newly minted version of rapamycin for use in the treatment of patients receiving renal transplants.[4] Boom. Welcome, to the family, Rapamune. Wyeth went a little overboard, peddling the rebadged Rapamune for all kinds of organ transplants and autoimmune assignments. Sales spiked, with 90 percent coming from off-label use other than renal transplants. Tumor killer, organ savior, and moneymaker. Life was good in Jersey. Hey, it was the nineties.

Like some giant starfish coveting a tasty oyster, Pfizer slowly crept closer to Wyeth and eventually couldn't resist the urge to merge. It pounced just as the FDA was closing the circle on the makers of Rapamune for illegally expanding the scope of the drug. In a colossal deal, Pfizer bought out Wyeth for $68 billion in 2009. Four years later, Pfizer-Wyeth was hammered for $490.9 million to close the chapter on years of outstanding federal and state civil and criminal claims over alleged product misrepresentation of Rapamune.[5] Hah, chump change. In 2013 alone, Pfizer made reported total sales of $51.6 billion, with a cool billion resulting from anti-tumor rapalogs alone. It's a good thing the extended rapamycin family has done well for itself. Pfizer spends a lot of time at the principal's office. They settled claims over the antipsychotic Geodon and the antibiotic Zyvox in 2010 for $2 billion. They closed out another federal lawsuit in 2016 for $784.6 million resulting from allegations of Medicaid fraud by Wyeth over Protonix, a popular stomach acid med.[6]

## THE JANUS MOLECULE

Ready for the plot twist? When scientists were studying the mechanism of rapamycin to tweak the drug for patentable spin-offs, they discovered something special.[7] Rapamycin attaches itself to a protein called FKB12, then gums up the receptors of a massive enzyme complex that functions at the nexus of cellular growth and metabolism. In 1991, they christened this beastly protein complex the mammalian (or mechanistic) target of rapamycin: mTOR (Figure 12). By any standard, mTOR is a big deal. It is made up of several large proteins that assemble as if they were a huge biologic transformer. Like the Roman god Janus, mTOR has two distinct faces.[8] When food resources are scarce and there aren't many amino acids around, mTOR floats around in the cytoplasm just chilling out like your basic friendly Autobot. When we're adults, this is good, since normal autophagy proceeds and tumors can't establish a beachhead.[9, 10] When mTOR gets lit up by a flood of amino acids or growth factors, it heads to the lysosomal surface, changes its conformation (shape), and starts phasing into full-on Decepticon battle mode. This starts a rapid cascade that kick-starts stem cell development, promotes cell proliferation, halts autophagy, and lets tumors run wild.[11] As it turns out, inhibiting this sprawling mTOR complex

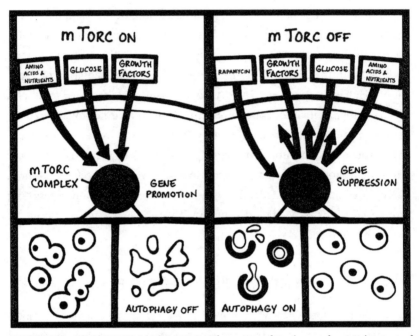

**FIGURE 12: THE JANUS MOLECULE.** The mammalian (or mechanistic) target of rapamycin complex (mTORC) is a sprawling protein metropolis that acts as a nutrient and growth factor sensor and control valve for cell growth. Its activity influences every aspect of metabolism and aging. When stimulated by plentiful resources or growth signals, mTORC turns on genes, makes proteins, pushes stem cell differentiation, and turns off autophagy. Growth goes wild and stem cells are exhausted (bad for aging). When nutrients are low (as in fasting, calorie restriction, or time-restricted feeding) or the receptors are blocked by drugs like rapamycin, mTORC turns off and autophagy proceeds, genes are suppressed, and protein synthesis slows. Growth is normal and stem cell reserves build (good for aging). (*Illustration: Jacob Scheyder*)

(mTORC) shape shifter with rapamycin disables many of the hallmarks of aging and increases longevity.[12, 13, 14]

There are two distinct kinds of mTORC, one that lines the lysosomes of cells when activated, mTORC1, and another, more mysterious version, mTORC2, that helps control the cytoskeleton and membrane permeability of cells.[15] When it senses sufficient amino acid resources or is stimulated by IGF-1, mTORC1 initiates protein production and using ATP for energy. It uses phosphorylation like chemical fingers to push and pull genetic buttons and levers as it coordinates growth on a genetic typewriter. High levels of ATP need to be present for proteins to be made. When activated, mTORC1 will keep pushing stem cells to differentiate until the lines are exhausted.

**TRIPLE THREAT**
Rapamycin and its rapalog descendants are named for their mysterious origins on Easter Island. They work as powerful immunosuppressants and tumor killers, and they might be future life extenders. These drugs work by blocking mTORC receptors.

Suppression of mTORC1 by rapamycin and rapalogs creates a receptor blockage that can slow down many of the metabolic penalties of aging. Genetically varied mice given rapamycin had remarkable improvements in longevity and vitality. It increased life span by 14 percent in females and 9 percent in males.[16, 17] The large, multifaceted nature of mTORC1 allows it to be finely regulated in different pockets by many different proteins and compounds. This allows it to influence many different physiologic functions instead of simply working as a growth valve and diverter. This is how rapalogs can simultaneously increase autophagy, increase senolytic clearance, improve energy reserves, slow down stem cell differentiation, and improve metabolic efficiency. Animal trials have shown improvement in cognition, nerve function, osteoporosis, inflammation, insulin sensitivity, mitochondrial function, and pulmonary fibrosis.[18, 19] These drugs have been used to coat cardiac stents to diminish restenosis rates. Two dueling rapalogs, Temsirolimus (aka Torisel from Pfizer) and Everolimus (aka Afinitor from Novartis), selectively block mTORC1 in the treatment of potentially lethal renal cancers, and the outlook is encouraging for breast cancer treatment.[20, 21]

Calibration is a beautiful thing when it comes to a medication. Rapalogs affect the immune system in a very dose-dependent fashion. Lower doses have minimal effects on immune function and have been well tolerated in animal studies and short-term human trialing.[22, 23] Low-dose cyclic treatment is shaping up as the best tactic for upcoming human rapalog longevity and health span trials. Higher doses will continue to be useful therapeutically for controlled immunosuppression and can effectively prevent solid organ transplant rejection.

Many more trials await rapalogs before their true risk-to-benefit ratio can be established in managing aging. Before you have an epiphany and embark on a life-affirming venture to Easter Island to slather yourself in moai mold, you could try less dramatic ways to naturally regulate your mTOR. Many bioactive flavonoids and polyphenols found in fruits and vegetables can help blunt the effects of mTORC. Coffee, tea, and caffeine all have modest roles in keeping mTORC in check. Exercise and time-restricted eating are also a cheaper way to push the candy-like red MTORC anti-aging button than buying a one-way ticket to the Hanga Roa Hilton.

## PATENT PENDING

Billions of dollars have a way of focusing the efforts of science. The race to find drugs to ease the burden of old age and help us die another day is taking researchers down increasingly bizarre paths. One of these twisty bends heads straight through our sensory receptors. We have evolved sophisticated sensory systems to monitor our environment and energy resources. Sight, sound, vibration, smell, pain, temperature, and pressure all provide crucial information for survival. The linkage between our senses and our metabolism is well established. Scientists are now looking at ways to manipulate sensory receptors to improve longevity.[24]

A pain receptor called TRPV-1 is particularly notable because when it's activated, it secretes a protein called CGRP that blocks insulin release and dulls metabolism, both enemies of longevity. TRPV-1, also known as the capsaicin receptor, is a cation gate in cellular membranes that regulates temperature, detects high heat, and transmits pain. TRPV-1 signaling in the hypothalamus links pain sensors to metabolic shifts. As we age, chronic inflammation leads to heightened TRPV-1 activation and decreased CGRP-mediated insulin secretion from the pancreas. The neurons are very sensitive to environmental stress both at the cellular and organ levels. Selective inhibition of TRPV-1 enhances longevity.[25, 26] Scientists at the University of California at Berkeley and the Salk Institute filed patents for this new class of potential longevity drugs within weeks of publication of their findings.

A new breed of scientists is examining the inner workings of our microbiome for answers to the riddles of aging. A group of microbiologists at Atlanta's Emory University is studying bacteria that secrete small bioactive peptides called indoles, like those found in certain plants and vegetables.[27] These bacteria and their indoles are found in many animals and change in character with aging. Copying these indoles may provide the source of a whole new class of pharmaceuticals to improve reproductive health, metabolism, and health span. If you want to see what most indoles look like, go stare at a head of broccoli, a food containing high concentrations of its own version of the stuff. Okay, don't stare at broccoli—that would just be weird.

We have covered a lot of ground in *The Fountain,* from the first hints of health and longevity in some of the most rugged and isolated places on Earth, the blue zones, to the inner workings of our vibrant and effervescent DNA. From the wonders of metabolism, to the dirty work of exercise and diet, we have sought ways to live better and longer. Ending in the lap of science, where questions far outnumber answers, we found ourselves once again scouring the edges of the planet and the depths of our bodies for answers to aging's riddles. Let's take one more look at what we do know about life and living. Hey, I don't want this date to ever end.

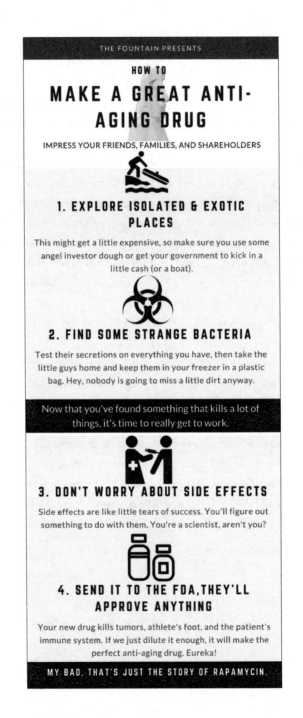

THE FOUNTAIN PRESENTS

**HOW TO**

# MAKE A GREAT ANTI-AGING DRUG

IMPRESS YOUR FRIENDS, FAMILIES, AND SHAREHOLDERS

## 1. EXPLORE ISOLATED & EXOTIC PLACES

This might get a little expensive, so make sure you use some angel investor dough or get your government to kick in a little cash (or a boat).

## 2. FIND SOME STRANGE BACTERIA

Test their secretions on everything you have, then take the little guys home and keep them in your freezer in a plastic bag. Hey, nobody is going to miss a little dirt anyway.

Now that you've found something that kills a lot of things, it's time to really get to work.

## 3. DON'T WORRY ABOUT SIDE EFFECTS

Side effects are like little tears of success. You'll figure out something to do with them. You're a scientist, aren't you?

## 4. SEND IT TO THE FDA, THEY'LL APPROVE ANYTHING

Your new drug kills tumors, athlete's foot, and the patient's immune system. If we just dilute it enough, it will make the perfect anti-aging drug. Eureka!

MY BAD, THAT'S JUST THE STORY OF RAPAMYCIN.

# PHASE FIVE
## THE PLAN

# 17

# THE FOUNTAIN PLAN

"If it could only be like this always—always summer."
—EVELYN WAUGH, BRIDESHEAD REVISITED, 1945

TIME TO WRAP IT up, folks. Don't worry, you don't have to take some sketchy *Cosmo*-like food personality quiz or sign up for a subscription to my monthly newsletter to find out what advice the science of aging has for you. Besides, if it all works out right, you'll live a lot longer and that will leave us plenty of time to hawk all sorts of longevity swag later. Right now, let's just focus on the core messages of *The Fountain* so you can start living a longer and healthier life right now.

## SCIENCE

Energy and error. If there is one thing you need to remember about aging, it's that it is embedded in a web of metabolism. This unified vision of how we age drives every element of intervention intended to improve health and longevity. The mitochondria, our unicellular overlords and oldest allies, provide the energy we need to live while we provide the shelter and resources they require.

Scientific research shows us that healthy aging hinges on maintaining sufficient reservoirs of energy and limiting the amount of errors that occur during the normal life cycles of our cells. Diet, exercise, and disease are entwined through very physical intermediaries like mMTOR and insulin receptors. Remember the seven hallmarks of aging: DNA damage, eroded telomeres, epigenetic alterations, mitochondrial dysfunction, nutrient-sensing deregulation, loss of proteostasis, and cellular senescence. All these roads eventually lead to breakdowns in intracellular communication and stem cell exhaustion. You don't burn out, you just run out of gas.

Every minute of every day, the DNA that carries the code for our lives is constantly changing in response to environmental signals. It is a vibrant dialogue. Although we are not genetic prisoners, we are certainly not completely free. We are constantly making choices. Good choices can maximize our health and longevity. Bad ones can quicken the pace of disease and energy demand. Every time we make a choice, or fail to choose how we want to live, we lose a little more freedom. Epigenetics is serious business. If you beat up your DNA, it can be difficult to recover. More importantly, poor decisions don't just affect you; they can be passed down to the next generation.

Similarly, making good choices in how you live, whether it is by exercising, managing stress, improving your diet, or simply through finding purpose, can repair and heal much of the lingering damage of your genetic legacy. I think of it like atoning for chromosomal original sin. I'm a Roman Catholic, so guilt is no stranger to me. Your DNA changes so quickly, so much, and so often that telomeric length appears to be elastic. It can change in length radically from day to day. Telomeres do have a Goldilocks zone where they are right-sized and your health is optimized. Too long and certain cancers can take hold. Too short and cell death becomes imminent. Tracking your telomeric lengths won't ensure longevity but could give you a barometer to figure out your general level of genomic stability and fitness.

We are finally figuring out that we are not the captains of our own ships. The rule of mitochondria is subtle but complete. Scientific research is finally providing us with a much more nuanced view of the inner workings of our complicated relationship with our ancestral visitors. New work provides evidence that the mitochondria are quite adept at dealing with the free radical wastes of energy production and use hydrogen peroxide to effectively regulate it.[1] Mitochondria are a libertine lot of royals, much more mobile and active than ever previously thought. They freely motor around the nucleoplasm, communicating and mixing their genetic material promiscuously with their neighbors. True symbiotes, mitochondria require payment for services rendered. It takes energy to make energy, and they fight for NAD+ with other heavy energy hogs, like the PARP-class DNA-repair enzymes. The mitochondria recycle their NAD+, but PARPs don't. There are 17 different kinds of PARPs, and they burn through NAD+ faster than a rookie running back going through a signing bonus. Mitochondria may have been the first unicellular organisms to hitch a ride on the human train, but they were not the last.

> **THE 300 TRILLION**
>
> The future of diet and medicine may lie in our microbiome. The bacteria that line our intestines and skin have a tremendous impact on our nutrition and general health. Optimizing this blend of passengers is becoming an important aspect in the diagnosis and treatment of many disorders, including diabetes and cancer.

Our bodies are coated with more than 300 trillion hitchhikers, and many have important roles in our metabolic ecosystem. We are finally starting to see the importance of our gut flora in how we eat, exercise, and live. Fine-tuning our microbiome and learning how to leverage it for better health and nutrition has become a new focus of research and corporate funding. We are truly entering a new era of personalized medicine, where individual genetic and microbiomic profiles will determine many aspects of our future health and well-being. Inner space has arrived.

## DIET

Whether you are a carnivore, omnivore, vegan, or vegetarian with tendencies, you need to learn where the holes exist in your diet and how to fill them to stay healthy. Vegans really need to watch their vitamin shortfalls. Vitamin B$_{12}$ and iron deficiencies are common among the leafy set. When it comes to food, vegans do have an important lesson for the epicurious among us. A plant-based diet provides a substantial base to build a good life on. Sorry, but potato chips do not count as a plant-based diet.

Meat eaters aren't off the hook, either. They need to watch their protein levels as they age. A diet high in protein can wreak havoc on the kidneys. Reining in protein intake will help keep IGF-1 below the cancer promotion levels. After 50, we really need to shift to a lower, more selective consumption of protein. If all goes well and you breach the age 80 tidal mark, going back to a higher-protein diet can help keep some meat on your bones. There is more vitamin D deficiency today than at any time since the Industrial Revolution. Everybody needs vitamin D$_3$ supplements for metabolic vitality, to support bone health, and to bundle up bands of circulating rogue IGF-1 and keep them from inciting a cancerous rebellion. Some supplements like fish oil are beat-up derivative substitutes that are merely the shadows of things that they shouldn't replace—like fish in your diet.

Some things aren't quite as bad as some people want you to believe. Sugar and salt are not weapons of mass destruction. They are not part of some unholy plot to undermine Western civilization. Sugar does not cause diabetes, and salt does not cause hypertension. In moderation.

Obesity is the real killer. Do you need to start watching the amount of sugar and salt in your diet? Yes. But the devil is in the details. Most of the extra salt and sugar of concern is in processed foods. It is a whole lot easier to avoid the dangerous processed meats and snacks now instead of battling obesity, hypertension, and diabetes later. If you stick to real food, you will be just fine. Well, if salt and sugar are fine, then fat must be bad. *Au contraire, mon frere.* The diet-heart hypothesis is baloney. Literally. Saturated fats do not cause elevated blood levels of cholesterol. Heart disease is an inflammatory disease driven by senescent cells that cause inflammation. Call it the pus-heart hypothesis instead, if you want. The bottom line is that you need some cholesterol to make things like testosterone to do things you like. Like sex. Omelets are in again, and real men can still eat quiche. Listen, if you have sky-high cholesterol and you don't eat fried lard, you probably have a genetic enzyme deficiency. Maybe you need a statin or other medication. Talk to your doctor. We still do that.

Gluten-free? Well, at least now you know what the hell gluten really is. Reminder: It's a water-catalyzed composite of proteins called glutenin and gliadin. They form a stretchy exoskeleton around starch molecules in wheat and other grains. When yeast is added to this hydro-elastic mix, the fungi get busy and digest the starch. This fermentation process of yeast produces carbon dioxide. The stretchy exoskeleton of gluten traps this, and the bread rises. In sourdough, there can be 100 times more bacteria than yeast. When they go ferment sugars like maltose, lactic acid is produced, giving the bread its slightly sour taste.

If you're gluten-free, you probably have rice flour tapping out wheat flour in a lot of your meals. This can cause problems since rice tends to bioaccumulate arsenic and mercury contaminants, which can lead to subtle heavy metal poisoning.[2] The number of gluten-sensitives and celiacs in the United States is far less than the number living the La Vida Sin Gluten. Keep going and you might give the vegans a run for their money. Don't look at me like that, you can't have my pizza.

The world's best dietary supplements may be coffee and tea. The flavonoids and polyphenols present in these brews can help pull your mTOR kill switch into the off position and maybe even keep you sane just a little longer. The caffeine is simply a bonus.

Hurt yourself? Fractures and sprains demand attention. Adding 500 milligrams of vitamin C and 1,500 milligrams of calcium to your diet while recovering can help you get a good result. No co-pay necessary. What about resveratrol? It did up my wine intake, but it proved disappointing as a cancer killer and longevity enhancer. It now has a more potent stepchild called pterostilbene with improved potency and bioavailability that might be worth a serious look for the daily rotation.[3]

Another supplement on the must-have short list: NAD-precursors. NAD+ is used through metabolism for electron chain transport of electrons to make ATP. The activity of most enzymes is determined by their shape.

NAD+ fills pockets on the surfaces of proteins, like the powerful PARP-class DNA-repair enzymes, like a battery cartridge to help them bind to their target and power chemical reactions. When NAD+ reserves are low, other proteins can fill these empty spots like they are playing microcellular musical chairs. David Sinclair's research group at Harvard Medical School has studied one of these opportunistic players, a protein called *deleted in breast cancer 1* (DBC1).[4] DBC1 fills the pocket on PARP1, and this blocks its ability to attach to the damaged DNA sequences that cause breast cancer. If you have a lot of NAD+ around, the pockets get filled by NAD+, DBC1 gets locked out, and PARP1 can do its job and fix the broken DNA strand. Once your NAD+ reservoir is exhausted, DBC1 and other proteins like it fill the voids. DNA damage accumulates, and it is a cancer coin-flip. Since maintenance of NAD+ reservoirs is also a crucial requirement for mitochondrial oxidative phosphorylation, ATP production, and DNA repair by PARP1, it makes sense to feed the energy pipeline. Nicotinamide riboside (NR) is the current NAD+ precursor of choice until more direct supplements become available.

## EXERCISE

When it comes to living longer, there is no pill, supplement, or exotic therapy as effective as daily exercise. Whether it's cardio, resistance, or a sublime blend, daily workouts are a key component of healthy living. Scientists have even put a number on it. For every minute of moderate to intense exercise after 40, you can expect 7 minutes of extra life.[5] Note: Thinking about exercise does not count.

What exercise is best? Since most exercise programs freely mix different disciplines, it can be a tough call. My preference is a HIIT program like P90X or my man Shaun T's T25 series because of their variety and intensity. If you're the competitive type, you might like CrossFit. Life in the Box is not as crazy as you think if you modify, modify, modify. If you are still a little timid about embarking on a HIIT training regimen, I would try to shoot for an hour of cardio 3 to 4 days a week. This could be running, swimming, biking, walking, elliptical (boring), or spinning. Weights and resistance training are important for building muscle and keeping your mitochondria happy. Once again, an hour per session is optimal, and you're looking at doing this twice a week.

I thought I would never be saying this, but I will anyway. Yoga or tai chi should be an integral part of your exercise program. One hour a week will fulfill your commitment. For older folks, the resistance elements of yoga, tai chi, and other variations of qigong martial arts can be a beautiful way to build muscle. That leaves 1 day a week for rest, reflection, and meditation. And sex. Don't forget sex. Probably dividing up the hour throughout the week on that one. It's not on the exercise list, but if it burns calories, it counts. Don't worry if you're not that active—thinking about sex counts as meditation.

Can you lose weight through exercise? Oh, you might lose a little in the beginning, but your body's evolutionary energy thermostat will fight you every step of the way. You're much better off controlling your weight by cutting calories and using time-restricted feeding to get rid of the gut. No time to work out? Make time. Seriously, just get moving. The benefits have far less to do with your weight than with your genetic fitness. Exercise works to improve all seven of the metabolic hallmarks of aging. Nothing else does.

## DRUGS

Can hormone replacement help you live longer? No, but it could help you live better. The Women's Health Initiative provided data on thousands of American women and how they responded to estrogen treatment. Although the study was halted prematurely due to concerns of heart disease and stroke, it provided a wealth of information that is still being interpreted. One group originally overlooked when the data was combed was young women with recent hysterectomy. They lived longer when given estrogen replacement therapy soon after the onset of menopause. If you are a woman nearing menopause or have had a hysterectomy, you need to give low-dose estrogen treatment a good long look. If you have had breast cancer, especially estrogen receptor-positive breast cancer, or you're at high genetic risk for breast cancer, then I would keep a wide berth of straight-up estrogen supplementation and think about other alternatives, like selective serotonin reuptake inhibitors that can ease the symptoms of menopause. Their dual nature as retooled antidepressants also provides the bonus of making the world look a little brighter.

Men also can benefit from hormone replacement. Low on T? Testosterone, an androgenic hormone, drops precipitously after adolescence. Modern society is also rough on the man juice, and research shows that levels in men in New England have dropped a lot over the past few years.[6,7] No comments, please. After all, I am a man from Nantucket. In cases where testosterone is low, supplementation makes sense. No increased risk for prostate cancer has been reported.

Growth hormone level is linked to our old friend IGF-1. Growth hormone drops dramatically as we age. This is good because it is a direct trigger for the duplicitous mTORC1 tumor promoter. Increasing GH increases IGF-1. You need to be careful when messing around with GH. It does help make more lean body mass, but it also increases the risk of diabetes, tumors, and heart disease. The big challenge with GH is getting a handle on accurately measuring levels in the body so we can better track the results of intervention. Despite all the issues hanging around GH use, if I could have half the guns of Stallone when I'm 70, I still might give it some serious consideration.

The most interesting hormone is oxytocin. Its rejuvenating effects on muscle are fascinating, and it may have even broader influence on metabolism and aging. As we get older, oxytocin levels begin to fall both peripherally and in the brain. Muscle atrophy and osteoporosis ensue. Feelings of loneliness and anxiety increase and can even become unmanageable. Research indicates that oxytocin influences vitality more than it does longevity. Oxytocin loss, through decreased production or failure of its transport protein, neurophysin, may be the real cause behind the frailty experienced by many elderly folks.[8] This could be a real breakthrough because it is the susceptibility to disease and injury that makes the final decade of life dangerous enough to warrant hazard pay. Can you buy liquid love? Not yet. Just like growth hormone, oxytocin is a controlled substance and is not available as a legal supplement. The potential that oxytocin has for decreasing some of the real physical risks of aging due to falls and fractures makes it a prime target of longevity research.

∞

I told you at the beginning that I was more afraid of living than dying. I am determined to not stand idly by as my body gradually fails and my mind slowly unravels. Neither should you. The lessons of *The Fountain* are clear. I have curated the most current scientific evidence to back them up. Eat a sensible, plant-based, calorie-controlled diet limited to 12 hours or less a day. Use supplements tactically to address specific shortfalls in your diet or lifestyle. NAD+ precursors, like NR, could help keep your energy tanks topped off and slow down some of the hallmarks of aging. Exercise as intensely as you can for an hour daily. Set aside time to just *think*. Get comfortable with silence and get your damn sleep. Find and embrace a raison d'être. Do something that interests you every day. Find humor in the commonplace. Be heroic. Fall in love.

In the end, quality of life trumps longevity. If you take care of your body, your mind, and your family, you will craft a life worth living no matter how much time you're given.

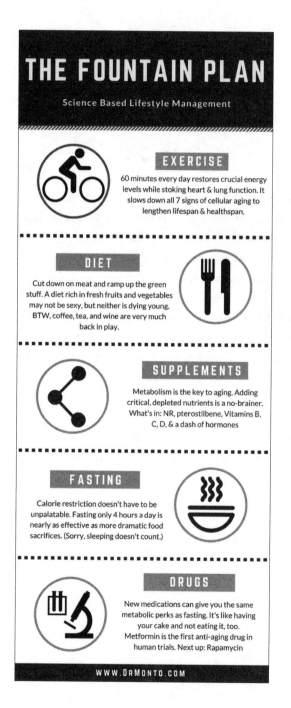

# THE FOUNTAIN PLAN

Science Based Lifestyle Management

**EXERCISE**

60 minutes every day restores crucial energy levels while stoking heart & lung function. It slows down all 7 signs of cellular aging to lengthen lifespan & healthspan.

**DIET**

Cut down on meat and ramp up the green stuff. A diet rich in fresh fruits and vegetables may not be sexy, but neither is dying young. BTW, coffee, tea, and wine are very much back in play.

**SUPPLEMENTS**

Metabolism is the key to aging. Adding critical, depleted nutrients is a no-brainer. What's in: NR, pterostilbene, Vitamins B, C, D, & a dash of hormones

**FASTING**

Calorie restriction doesn't have to be unpalatable. Fasting only 4 hours a day is nearly as effective as more dramatic food sacrifices. (Sorry, sleeping doesn't count.)

**DRUGS**

New medications can give you the same metabolic perks as fasting. It's like having your cake and not eating it, too. Metformin is the first anti-aging drug in human trials. Next up: Rapamycin

WWW.DRMONTO.COM

# ACKNOWLEDGMENTS

**NEVER HAVE SO MANY** done so much for so few.

I want to thank everyone who made *The Fountain* possible, but especially:

- Bill Maher, for proving that integrity, honesty, and loyalty are the true measures of success.
- My uber-agent, Alan Morell of Creative Management Partners, for turning his idea for this project into my obsession.
- My brother, Mark Monto, for keeping common sense alive in Hollywood.
- My son, Alex Monto, for whatever magic he wielded to make me look good on film.
- My talented young illustrator, Jacob Scheyder, for making the complex science behind *The Fountain* soft and cuddly.
- The literary goddesses of Rodale Books: Maria Rodale, Gail Gonzales, Jennifer Levesque, Marisa Vigilante, Brianne Sperber, Emily Eagan, Aly Mostel, Danielle Curtis, and my awesome editors, Shannon Welch and Amy Kovalski, for taking a chance on a first-time author and believing in my vision.

- Bert Ulrich, Connie Moore, and all the folks at NASA, for making space cool again.
- Everyone at Nantucket Cottage Hospital, for making me a better doctor and restoring my faith in medicine.
- My patients, for trusting me to always do the right thing for them.

# GLOSSARY

**ADP:** adenosine diphosphate, a nucleotide that combines with a phosphate to form ATP to store energy for cellular metabolism

**ALLELE:** alternate versions of the same gene

**ANAEROBIC:** process that occurs in the absence of oxygen

**APOPTOSIS:** preprogrammed cell death

**ARED:** Active Resistive Exercise Device; a strength-training machine designed by NASA for use in weightless environments

**ATOM:** the smallest stable piece of matter; it is made up of protons and neutrons

**ATP:** adenosine triphosphate; splits off a phosphate molecule in a process that produces energy for cellular metabolism

**AUTOPHAGY:** natural, regulated cell destruction and recycling process

**BACTERIA:** microscopic, single-cell organisms that thrive in diverse environments

**BIOELECTRIC:** theory that the body uses innate electrical fields and currents to direct development, healing, and aging

**CELL:** the smallest, most fundamental unit of an organism; typically contains cytoplasm surrounding a nucleus

**CENTROMERE:** condensed zones of DNA that divide the chromosomes into short (p) and long (q) arms to form an x-shape

**CHAPERONE:** proteins that pick up and guide misfolded or damaged proteins to recycling or autophagic zones

**CHROMATIN:** solenoid-shaped strands of DNA, histone proteins, and mRNA

**CHROMOSOME:** threadlike strands of tightly wound DNA within the nucleus

**COMPOUND:** combination of atoms of different types (for example, glucose is a compound made up of carbon, hydrogen, and oxygen, or $C_6H_{12}O$)

**CONCENTRIC EXERCISE:** muscular contraction with muscle shortening

**CRISPRCAS9:** Clustered Regularly Interspaced Short Palindromic Repeats

**DNA:** deoxyribonucleic acid; a twisting triple helical structure made up of amino acids that carries all the genetic instructions for cells

**ECCENTRIC EXERCISE:** muscular contraction with muscle extension

**ELECTROLYTES:** elements that release ions when they break apart in water ($NaCL + H_2O = Na(+)$ and $CL(-)$)

**ELECTRON:** negatively charged particles without mass that form a cloud around the nucleus of an atom

**ENZYME:** protein catalyst produced by cells to drive chemical reactions

**EPIGENETICS:** the study of how environmental stresses and interaction modify genetic expression

**ESTROGEN:** steroid hormone that regulates female characteristics

**GENE:** short DNA sequences that code for protein or physical traits

**GENETIC EXPRESSION:** the transcription of genetic information to mRNA and then protein production

**GEROSCIENCE:** a new field of translational science combining various scientific disciplines to study aging

**HISTONE:** proteins that bond to DNA, creating protective folds

**HORMONE:** regulatory substance produced to stimulate or regulate tissue functions

**HUMAN GROWTH HORMONE (GH):** a hormone produced by the pituitary gland that stimulates muscle and bone formation

INSULIN: a hormone produced in the pancreas by the islet of Langerhans that controls the amount of glucose in the blood

ION: an atom that has lost or gained electrons to become a charged particle (an atom that is positive or negative) capable of forming bonds

KINASE: an enzyme that transfers a phosphate group from ATP to a specific target

LYSOSOME: a cell organelle that is surrounded by a membrane, has an acidic interior, and contains hydrolytic enzymes that break down proteins and complex molecules

MACRONUTRIENTS: substances required in large amounts for growth and development (fats, carbohydrates, proteins, calcium, magnesium, potassium, etc.)

MDNA: mitochondrial DNA; unique genetic material present in mitochondria that combines with cellular host DNA for normal energy production

MEMBRANE: a microscopic double layer of lipids and proteins that bounds cells and organelles and forms structures within cells

METFORMIN: a drug marketed under the trade name Glucophage, used to control type 2 diabetes

METHYLATION: process that reversibly adds methyl groups to DNA to alter gene transcription

MICROBIOME: microorganisms in symbiosis with the body that help defend against infection, break down food, and produce vitamins

MICRONUTRIENTS: substances required in trace amounts for growth and development (vitamin B3, vitamin D3, vitamin E, zinc, selenium, etc.)

MITOCHONDRIA: organelles in cells that produce ATP (and energy) and have their own unique mDNA

MITOSIS: the copying and parceling of DNA and microtubules during cell division

MOLECULE: combinations of atoms of the same type

MTORC: mammalian (or mechanistic) target of rapamycin complex; a large conglomerate of multiple proteins that acts as a control valve for metabolic growth functions

NAD: nicotinamide adenine dinucleotide; molecule that binds with hydrogen in the mitochondria in the electron transport chain for energy production

NR: nicotinamide riboside; form of vitamin B3 that is a precursor to NAD

NUCLEUS: membrane-enclosed cellular command center containing chromosomes

ORGANELLE: a specialized structure within a cell

P53: sentinel protein that identifies chromosomes with damaged DNA

PROTEIN: nitrogen-based compound made up of long chains of amino acids to perform specific structures or tasks

PROTEOSTASIS: balancing the production, destruction, and recycling of system proteins for cellular health

PROTON PUMP: an integral membrane protein that moves protons across a membrane

RAPAMYCIN: a drug used to prevent rejection of organ and bone marrow transplant grafts with tumor-killing and possible anti-aging effects

RIBOSOME: complex molecular machine that produces proteins from RNA command

RNA: ribonucleic acid; translated from DNA codes to produce specific proteins

SENESCENCE: irreversible cellular growth arrest without death

SENOLYTICS: class of drugs designed to destroy senescent cells and inflammatory damage

SIRTUINS: a class of proteins that are involved in many metabolic processes and insulin regulation that may be activated by low-calorie stress periods

STEM CELL: undifferentiated cell that can give rise to many different cell types

TELOMERASE: an enzyme that helps maintain telomere length and prevent gradual shortening during sequential rounds of cellular division

TELOMERES: densely packed caps of repetitive DNA sequences that cap the ends of chromosomes and buffer against damage during cell division

VIRUS: ancient infectious microorganisms that invade cells and commandeer the production of foreign proteins

# ENDNOTES

## CHAPTER 1

1. Poulain M, Pes GM, Grasland C et al. Identification of a geographic area characterized by extreme longevity in the Sardinia Island: the AKEA study. *Experimental Gerontology* 2004;39(9):1423–9.

2. Buettner D. *The Blue Zone: Lessons for Living Longer from the People Who've Lived the Longest.* National Geographic Books, 2008.

3. Buettner D. *The Blue Zone Solution: Eating and Living like the World's Healthiest People.* National Geographic Books, 2015.

4. Lawrence DH. *Sea and Sardinia (1920).* Cambridge University Press, 1997.

5. https://www.theguardian.com/world/2016/aug/12/ethical-questions-raised-in -search-for-sardinian-centenarians-secrets

6. Poulain M et al. The AKEA study. *Experimental Gerontology* 2004.

7. Tognotti E. Program to eradicate malaria in Sardinia, 1946–1950. *Emerging Infectious Diseases*/CDC 2009;15(9):1460–6.

8. Tognotti E. Malaria in Sardinia, CDC 2009.

9. Steri M, Orru V, Idda ML et al. Overexpression of the cytokine BAFF and autoimmunity risk. *New England Journal of Medicine* 2017;376(17):1615–26.

10. Mydans, C. The Okinawa junk heap. *Life,* December 19, 1949, 27(25).

11. Bernstein AM, Willcox DC, Tamaki H et al. First autopsy study of an Okinawan

centenarian: absence of many age-related diseases. *Journal of Gerontology* 2004;59A(11): 1195–9.

12. Willcox DC, Willcox BJ, He Q et al. They really are that old: A validation study of centenarian prevalence in Okinawa. *Journal of Gerontology* 2008;63A(4): 338–49.

13. Willcox BJ, Willcox DC, Curb JD et al. Siblings of Okinawan centenarians share lifelong mortality advantages. *Journal of Gerontology* 2006;61(4):345–54.

14. Kerr GH. *Okinawa: The Story of an Island People.* Tuttle Publishing, 2011.

15. Willcox DC, Willcox BJ, Hsueh WC et al. Genetic determinants of exceptional human longevity: Insights from the Okinawa centenarian study. *Age* 2006;28(4):313–32.

16. Oscar Wilde (quote c1900).

17. Papalas AJ. *Ancient Ikaria.* Balchazy-Carducci Publishers, 1992.

18. Georgirenes J. *A Description of the Present State of Samos, Nikaria, Patmos, and Mount Athos* (1677), London, 54–70.

19. Panagiotakos DB, Chrysohoou C, Siasos G et al. Sociodemographic and lifestyle statistics of oldest old people (>80 years) living in Ikaria island: the Ikaria study. *Cardiology Research and Practice* 2011;2(24):679187.

20. Pittier H. Impresiones y recuerdos: Es posiblemente el primer testimonio sobre la exceptional longevidad de los habitantes de la Peninsula de Nicoya, Costa Rica. *Pandemonium* 2011;3(45):5–8.

21. Rosero-Bixby L: The exceptionally high life expectancy of Costa Rican nonagenarians. *Demography* 2008;45(3):673–91.

22. Rosero-Bixby L, Dow WH, Rehkopf DH. The Nicoyan region of Costa Rica: a high longevity island for elderly males. *Vienna Yearbook of Population Research* 2013;11:109–36.

23. Rehkopf DH, Dow WH, Rosero-Bixby L et al. Longer leukocyte telomere length in Costa Rica's Nicoya Peninsula: a population-based study. *Experimental Gerontology* 2013;48(11):1266–73.

24. McEwen LM, Morin AM, Edgar RD et al. Differential DNA methylation and lymphocyte proportions in a Costa Rican high longevity region. *Epigenetics & Chromatin* 2017;10(21).

25. http://www.iret.una.ac.cr/

26. Wessling C, Castillo L, Elinder CG. Pesticide poisonings in Costa Rica. *Scandinavian Journal of Work, Environment & Health* 1993;19(4):227–35.

27. Shavlik DJ, Fraser GE. Ten years of life: is it a matter of choice? *Archives of Internal Medicine* 2001;13(161):1645–52.
28. Orlich MJ, Singh PN, Sabate J, et al. Vegetarian dietary patterns and mortality in Adventist Health Study 2. *JAMA Internal Medicine* 2013;173:1230–8.
29. Orzlowska E, Jacobson JJ, Bareh GM et al. Food intake diet and sperm characteristics in a blue zone: a Loma Linda Study. *European Journal of Obstetrics & Gynecology and Reproductive Biology* 2016;5:43.

## CHAPTER 2

1. https://www.nasa.gov/twins-study
2. Blackpurn E, Epel E. *The Telomere Effect.* Grand Central Publishing, 2017.
3. Rivera T, Haggblom C, Cosconati S et al. A balance between elongation and trimming regulates telomere stability in stem cells. *Nature Structural & Molecular Biology* 2017;24:30–9.
4. Horvath S, Lu AT, Mah V et al. The cerebellum ages slowly according to the epigenetic clock. *Aging* 2015;7(5):294–305.
5. Bianconi E, Piovesan A, Faccin F et al. An estimation of the number of cells in the human body. *Annals of Human Biology* 2013;40(6):463–71.
6. Pray L. Discovery of DNA structure and function: Watson and Crick. *Nature Education* 2008;1(1):100.
7. Crisp A, Boschetti C, Perry M et al. Expression of multiple horizontally acquired genes is a hallmark of both vertebrate and invertebrate genomes. *Genome Biology* 2015;16:50.
8. Joehanes R, Just AC, Marioni RE et al. Epigenetic signatures of cigarette smoking. *Circulation* 2016;9:436–47.
9. Ou HD, Phan S, Deerinck TJ et al. ChromET: visualizing 3D chromatin structure and compaction in interphase and mitotic cells. *Science* 2017;357(6349):370.
10. Graham JE, Marians KJ, Kowalczykowski SC. Independent and stochastic action of DNA polymerases in the ribosome. *Cell* 2017;169(7):1201–13.
11. López-Otín C, Galluzzi L, Freije JMP et al. Metabolic control of longevity. *Cell* 2016; 166:802–21.
12. Nguyen NM, de Oliveira Andrade F, Jin L et al. Maternal intake of high n-9 polyunsaturated fatty acid diet during pregnancy causes transgenerational increase in mammary cancer risk in mice. *Breast Cancer Research* 2017;19:77–109.

13. Thompson JR, Vaileau JC, Barling AN et al. Exposure to a high-fat diet during early development programs behavior and impairs the central serotonergic system in juvenile non-human primates. *Frontiers in Endocrinology* 2017;7:1–38.

14. Furman D, Chang J, Lartigue L et al. Expression of specific inflammasome gene modules stratified older individuals into two extreme clinical and immunological states. *Nature Medicine* 2017;23:174–84.

15. Levine ME, Suarez JA, Brandhorst S et al. Low protein intake is associated with a major reduction in IGF-1, cancer, and overall mortality in the 65 and younger but not older population. *Cell Metabolism* 2014;19(3):407–17.

16. Baker DJ, Childs BG, Durik M et al. Naturally occurring p16(Ink4a)-positive cells shorten healthy lifespan. *Nature* 2016;530:184–204.

17. Zhang Y, Kim MS, Jian B et al. Hypothalamic stem cells control ageing speed partly through exosomal miRNAs. *Nature* 2017;548(7665):52–57.

## CHAPTER 3

1. Latorre-Pellicer A, Morano-Loshuartos R, Lechuga-Vieco A et al. Mitochondrial and nuclear DNA matching shapes metabolism and healthy ageing. *Nature* 2016;535:561–65.

2. Lewis SC, Uchiyama F, Numan J. ER-mitochondria contacts couple mtDNA synthesis with mitochondrial division in human cells. *Science* 2016;353.

3. Singh B, Modica-Napolitano JS, Sigh KK. Defining the momiome: promiscuous information transfer by mobile mitochondria and mitochondrial genome. *Seminars in Cancer Biology* 2017;5(11).

4. Grimm A A, Eckart A. Brain ageing and neurodegeneration: from a mitochondrial point of view. *Journal of Neurochemistry* 2017;4(11).

5. Onyango IG, Khan SM, Bennett JP. Mitochondria in the pathophysiology of Alzheimer's and Parkinson's diseases. *Frontiers in Bioscience* 2017;1(22):854–72.

6. Munro D, Treberg JR. A radical shift in perspective: mitochondria as regulators of reactive oxygen species. *Journal of Experimental Biology* 2017;1(220):1170–80.

7. Willey C, Velarde MC, Lecot P et al. Mitochondrial dysfunction induces senescence with a discrete secretory phenotype. *Cell Metabolism* 2016;23(2):303–14.

8. Yang T, Sauve AA. NAD metabolism and sirtuins: metabolic regulation of protein deacetylation in stress and toxicity. *AAPS Journal* 2006;12(4).

9. Verdin E. NAD+ in aging, metabolism, and neurodegeneration. *Science* 2016;166:1208–13.

10. Fang EF, Scheibye-Knudson M, Cua KF et al. Nuclear DNA damage signaling to mitochondria in ageing. *Nature Reviews Molecular Cell Biology* 2016;308–21.

11. Ascher G, Garfield D, Stratmann M et al. SIRT1 regulates circadian clock gene expression through PERs deacetylation. *Cell* 2008;134(2):317–28.

12. Schweier MJ, Knudsen KE. Transcriptional roles of PARP-1 in cancer. *Molecular Cancer Research* 2014;12(8):1069–80.

13. Sahar S, Massubuchi S, Eckel-Mahan K et al. Circadian control of fatty acid elongation by SIRT1 protein-mediated deacetylation of acetyl-coenzyme A synthetase 1. *Journal of Biological Chemistry* 2014; 289:6091–97.

14. Canto C, Auwery J. Targeting SIRT1 to improve metabolism: all you need is NAD+? *Pharmacological Reviews* 2012;64(1):166–87.

15. Chang HC, Guarente L. SIRT1 mediates central circadian control in the SCN by a mechanism that decays with aging. *Cell* 2013;153:1448–60.

16. Gomes AP, Price NL, Ling AJ et al. Declining NAD+ induces a pseudohypoxic state disrupting nuclear-mitochondrial communication during aging. *Cell* 2013;155:1624–38.

## CHAPTER 4

1. McDonald RB, Ramsey JJ. Honoring Clive McCay and 75 years of calorie restriction research. *Journal of Nutrition* 2010;140(7):1204–10.

2. Hayashida S, Arimoto A, Kuramoto T et al. Fasting promotes the expression of SIRT1, an NAD+-dependent protein deacetylase, via activation of PPAP-alpha in mice. *Molecular and Cellular Biochemistry* 2010;339(1–2):285–92.

3. Madeo F, Zimmermann A, Maiuri MC et al. Essential role for autophagy in life span extension. *Journal of Clinical Investigation* 2015; 125:85–93.

4. López-Otín C, Blasco MA, Serrano M et al. The hallmarks of aging. *Cell* 2013;153(6):1194–217.

5. Kotas M, Gorecki MC, Gillum MP. Sirtuin-1 is a nutrient-dependent modulator of inflammation. *Adipocyte* 2013;2(2):113–18.

6. Wang A, Huen SC, Luan HH et al. Opposing effects of fasting metabolism on tissue tolerance in bacterial and viral inflammation. *Cell* 2016;166(6):1512–25.

7. Cheng CW, Villani V, Buono R et al. Fasting-mimicking diet promotes Ngn3-driven beta-cell regeneration to reverse diabetes. *Cell* 2017;168(5):775–88.

8. Fontana L, Villareal DT, Das SK et al. Effects of 2-year calorie restriction on circulating levels of IGF-1, IGF-binding proteins and cortisol in non-obese men and women: randomized clinical trial. *Cell* 2016;15(1):22–27.

9. Deng Y, Wang ZV, Gordillo R et al. An adipo-biliary-uridine axis that regulates energy homeostasis. *Science* 2017;355(6330):1124.

10. Trepanowski JF, Kroeger CM, Barnosky A. Effect of alternate-day fasting on weight loss, weight maintenance, and cardioprotection among metabolically healthy obese adults. *JAMA Internal Medicine* 2017;5.

11. Cheng CW et al. Fasting-mimicking diet. *Cell* 2017.

12. Ascher G, Sassone-Coral P. Time for food: the intimate interplay between nutrition, metabolism, and the circadian clock. *Cell* 2015;161:84–92.

13. Moro T, Tinsley G, Bianco A et al. Effects of eight weeks of time-restricted feeding (16/8) on basal metabolism, maximal strength, body composition, inflammation, and cardiovascular risk factors in resistance-trained males. *Journal of Translational Medicine* 2016;14:290.

14. Antoni R, Johnston KL, Collins AL et al. Effects of intermittent fasting on glucose and lipid metabolism. *Proceedings of the Nutrition Society* 2017;16:1–8.

15. Harvie M, Howell A. Potential benefits and harms of intermittent energy restriction and intermittent fasting amongst obese, overweight, and normal weight subjects—a narrative review of human and animal evidence. *Behavioral Sciences* 2017;7(4):1–22.

## CHAPTER 5

1. Lander ES. The Heroes of CRISPR. *Cell* 2015;164:18–28.

2. Datsenko KA, Pougach K, Tikhonov A et al. Molecular memory of prior infections activates the CRISPR/Cas adaptive bacterial immunity system. *Nature Communications* 2012;10(3):945.

3. Koonin EV, Krupovic M. Evolution of adaptive immunity from transposable elements combined with innate immune systems. *Nature Reviews* 2014;16:184–92.

4. Barrangou R, Fremaux C, Deveau H et al. CRISPR provides acquired resistance against viruses in prokaryotes. *Science* 2007;315:1709–12.

5. Jinek M, Chylinski K, Fonfara I et al. A programmable dual-RNA-guided DNA endonuclease in adaptive bacterial immunity. *Science* 2012;337(6096):816–21.

6. Shipman SL, Nivala J, Macklis JD et al. CRISPR-Cas encoding of a digital movie into the genomes of a population of living bacteria. *Nature* 2017;23017.

7. Kim K, Park SW, Kim JH et al. Genome surgery using Cas9 ribonucleoproteins for the treatment of age-related macular degeneration. *Genome Research* 2017;11.

8. Bengtsson NE, Hall JK, Odom GL et al. Muscle-specific CRISPR/cas9 dystrophin gene editing ameliorates pathophysiology in a mouse model for Duchenne muscular dystrophy. *Nature Communications* 2016;1–9.

9. Schaefer KA, Wu WH, Colgan DF et al. Unexpected mutations after CRISPR-Cas9 editing *in vivo*. *Nature Methods* 2017;14(6):547–48.

10. Waddington SN, Privolizzi R, Karda R et al. A broad overview and review of CRISPR-cas technology and stem cells. *Current Stem Cell Reports* 2016; 2:9-20.

11. De Ravin SS, Xi L, Wu X et al. CRISPR-Cas9 gene repair of hematopoietic stem cells from patients with X-linked chronic granulomatous disease. *Science Translational Medicine* 2017;9(37).

12. Takahashi K, Yamanaka S. Induction of pluripotent stem cells from mouse embryonic and adult fibroblast cultures by defined factors. *Cell* 2006;126(4):663–76.

13. Ocampo A, Reddy P, Martinez-Redondo A et al. In vivo amelioration of age-associated hallmarks by partial reprogramming. *Cell* 2016;167(7):1719–33.

14. National Academy of Sciences Human Gene Editing Report, Feb. 14, 2017.

15. Ma H, Marti-Gutierrez N, Park SW et al. Correction of a pathogenic gene mutation in human embryos. *Nature* 2017;548:413–19.

## CHAPTER 6

1. Ng M, Fleming T, Robinson M et al. Global, regional, and national prevalence of overweight and obesity in children and adults during 1980-2013: a systematic analysis for the Global Burden of Disease Study 2013. *Lancet* 2014;384(9945): 766–81.

2. Pontzer H, Raichlen DA, Wood BW et al. Hunter-gatherer energetics and human obesity. *PLOS One* 2012;1–10.

3. Fothergill E, Go J, Howard L et al. Persistent metabolic adaptation 6 years after "The Biggest Loser" competition. *Obesity* 2016;24:1612–19.

4. Thomas DM, Bouchard C, Church T et al. Why do individuals not lose more weight from an exercise intervention at a defined dose? An energy balance analysis. *Obesity Reviews* 2012;13(10):835–47.

5. Ungar P. The "true" human diet. *Scientific American* April 17, 2017, https://blogs .scientificamerican.com/guest-blog/the-true-human-diet/.

6. Mozaffarian D, Katan MB, Ascherio A et al. Trans fatty acids and cardiovascular disease. *New England Journal of Medicine* 2006;13(15):1601–13.

7. Taubes G. The soft science of dietary fat. *Science* 2001;291:2536–45.

8. Mann GV. Diet-heart: end of an era. *New England Journal of Medicine* 1977;297(12):644–50.

9. Frantz ID, Dawson E, Ashman PA et al. Test of effect of lipid lowering by diet on cardiovascular risk: the Minnesota coronary survey. *Arteriosclerosis* 1989;(9):129–35.

10. Ramsden CE, Zamora D, Majchrzak-Hong S et al. Re-evaluation of the traditional diet-heart hypothesis: analysis of recovered data from Minnesota Coronary Experiment (1968-1973). *British Medical Journal* 2016;353:1–17.

11. Kuipers RS, de Graaf DJ, Loxwolda MF et al. Saturated fats, carbohydrates, and cardiovascular disease. *Netherlands Journal of Medicine* 2011;69(9):372–78.

12. Ramsden CE, Zamora D, Leelarthaepin B et al. Use of dietary linoleic acid for secondary prevention of coronary heart disease and death: evaluation of recovered data from the Sydney Diet Heart Study and updated meta-analysis. *British Medical Journal* 2013;346.

13. de Souza RJ, Mente A, Morleanu A et al. Intake of saturated and trans unsaturated fatty acids and risk of all-cause mortality, cardiovascular disease, and type 2 diabetes: systematic review and meta-analysis of observational studies. *British Medical Journal* 2015;35.

14. Zong G, Li Y, Wanders AJ et al. Intake of individual saturated fatty acids and risk of coronary heart disease in US men and women: two prospective longitudinal cohort studies. *British Medical Journal* 2016;355:1–11.

15. Malhotra A, Redberg RF, Meier P. Saturated fat does not clog the arteries: coronary heart disease is a chronic inflammatory condition, the risk of which can be effectively reduced from healthy lifestyle interventions. *British Medical Journal* 2017;51(15):1111–12.

16. Kleber ME, Delgado GE, Lorkowski S et al. Trans-fatty acids and mortality in patients referred for coronary angiography: the Ludwigshafen risk and cardiovascular health study. *European Heart Journal* 2016;37(13):1072–78.

17. Estruch R, Ros E, Sala-Salvado J et al. Primary prevention of cardiovascular disease with a Mediterranean diet. *New England Journal of Medicine* 2013;368:1279–90.

18. Groopman J. Is fat killing you, or is sugar? *The New Yorker* April 3, 2017, http://www.newyorker.com/magazine/2017/04/03/is-fat-killing-you-or-is-sugar.

19. Hämäläinen E, Adlercreutz H, Puska P, Pietinen P. Diet and serum sex hormones in healthy men. *Journal of Steroid Biochemistry* 1984;20(1):459–64.

20. Volek JS, Kraemer WJ, Bush JA et al. Testosterone and cortisol in relationship to dietary nutrients and resistance exercise. *Journal of Applied Physiology* 1997;82(1):49–54.

21. Barber, Malcolm. *The Two Cities: Medieval Europe, 1050–1320* (2nd ed.). Routledge, 2004.

22. Ponting C. *World History: A New Perspective*. Chatto & Windus, London, 2001.

23. https://www.ers.usda.gov/topics/crops/sugar-sweeteners.aspx

24. Yudkin JA. *Pure, White, and Deadly: The Problem of Sugar.* Harper Collins, New York, 1972.

25. Taubes G. *The Case against Sugar.* Knopf, New York, 2016.

26. Guyenet S. Bad sugar or bad journalism? An expert review of "the case against sugar." Jan 26, 2017, http://www.stephanguyenet.com/bad-sugar-or-bad-journalism -an-expert-review-of-the-case-against-sugar/.

27. https://www.cdc.gov/nchs/data/hestat/obesity_adult_11_12/obesity_adult_11_12.pdf

28. Menke A, Casagrande S, Geiss L et al. Prevalence of and trends in diabetes among adults in the United States, 1988-2012. *JAMA* 2015:314(10):1021–29.

29. Hall KD. A review of the carbohydrate-insulin model of obesity. *European Journal of Clinical Nutrition* 2017;71(3):323–26.

30. Davegardh C, Broholm C, Perfilyev A et al. Abnormal epigenetic changes during differentiation of human skeletal muscle stem cells from obese subjects. *BMC Medicine* 2017;15:39.

31. Hamburg NM, McMacklin CJ, Huang AL et al. Physical inactivity rapidly induces insulin resistance and microvascular dysfunction in healthy volunteers. *Arteriosclerosis, Thrombosis, and Vascular Biology* 2007;27(12):2650–56.

32. Lozano I, Van der Werf R, Bietiger W et al. High-fructose and high-fat diet-induced disorders in rats: impact on diabetes risk, hepatic and vascular complications. *Nutrition & Metabolism* 2016;25:13–15.

33. Dobson AJ, Ezcurra M, Flanagan CE et al. Nutritional programming of lifespan by FOXO inhibition on sugar-rich diets. *Cell Reports* 2017;18(2):299–306.

34. Kitahara CM, Flint AJ, de Gonsalez AB et al. Association between class III obesity (BMI of 40–59 kg/m) and mortality: a pooled analysis of 20 prospective studies. *PLOS Medicine* July 8, 2014.

35. Stone TW, Darlington LG. Microbial carcinogenic toxins and anti-cancer protectants. *Cellular and Molecular Life Sciences* 2017;74(14):2627–43.

36. Roberts RO, Roberts LA, Geda YE et al. Relative intake of macronutrient impacts of mild cognitive impairment or dementia. *Journal of Alzheimer's Disease* 2012;32:329–39.

37. Moser VA, Poke C. Obesity accelerates Alzheimer-related pathology in APOE4 but not APOE3 mice. *eNeuro* 2017;4(3):1–18.

38. Fowler SPG, Williams K, Hazuda HP. Diet soda intake is associated with long-term increases in waist circumference in a biethnic cohort of older adults; the San Antonio longitudinal study of aging. *Journal of the American Geriatrics Society* 2015;63(4):708–15.

39. Chia CW, Shardell M, Tanaka T et al. Chronic low-calorie sweetener use and risk of abdominal obesity among older adults: a cohort study. *PLOS One* November 23, 2016,1–10.

40. Suez J, Korem T, Zeevi D et al. Artificial sweeteners induce glucose intolerance by altering the gut microbiota. *Nature* 2014;514(7521):181–86.

41. Pase MP, Himali JJ, Beiser AS et al. Sugar- and artificially sweetened beverages and the risks of incident stroke and dementia: a prospective cohort study. *Stroke* 2017;48:1139–46.

42. Wershing H, Gardener H, Sacco RL. Sugar-sweetened and artificially sweetened beverages in relation to stroke and dementia: are sugar drinks hard on the brain? *Stroke* 2017;48:1129–31.

43. https://www.scientificamerican.com/article/its-time-to-end-the-war-on-salt/

44. http://www.cochrane.org/CD009217/VASC_reduced-dietary-salt-prevention-cardiovascular-disease

45. O'Donnell M, Mente A, Ragarajan S et al. Urinary sodium and potassium excretion, mortality, and cardiovascular events. *New England Journal of Medicine* 2014;371:612–23.

46. Lelon H, Galan P, Kesse-Guyot E et al. Relationship between nutrition and blood pressure: a cross-sectional analysis from the NutriNet-Santé study, a French web-based cohort study. *American Journal of Hypertension* 2015;28(3):362–71.

47. Mente A, O'Donnell M, Ragarajan S et al. Associations of urinary sodium excretion with cardiovascular events in individuals with and without hypertension: a pooled analysis of data from four studies. *Lancet* 2016;388(1043):465–75.

48. Rakova N, Kitada K, Lerchl K et al. Increased salt consumption induces body water conservation and decreases fluid intake. *Journal of Clinical Investigation* 2017;127(5):1932–43.

49. Kitada K, Daub S, Zhang Y et al. High salt intake reprioritizes osmolyte and energy metabolism for body fluid conservation. *Journal of Clinical Investigation* 2017;127(5):1944–59.

50. Sharipova M, Balaban N, Kayumov A et al. The expression of the serine protease gene of *Bacillus intermedius* in *Bacillus subtilis*. *Microbiological Research* 2008;163:39–50.

51. Tsugane S, Sasazuki S, Kobayashi M et al. Salt and salted food intake and subsequent risk of gastric cancer among middle-aged Japanese men and women. *British Journal of Cancer* 2004;90:128–34.

52. Leonard MM, Camhi S, Huedo-Medina TB et al. Celiac disease genomic, environ-mental, microbiome, and metabolomic (CDGEMM) study design: approach to the future of personalized prevention of celiac disease. *Nutrients* 2015;7(11):9325–36.

53. Vocke G. Wheat's role in the US diet has changed over the decades. ER/USDA briefing room, 2009, http://www.ers.usda.gov/topics/crops/wheat/whetats-role-in -the-us-diet.aspx.

54. Kasarda DD. Can an increase in celiac disease be attributed to an increase in the gluten content of wheat as a consequence of wheat breeding? *Journal of Agricul-tural and Food Chemistry* 2013;61(6):1155–59.

55. Perlmutter D. *Grain Brain: The Surprising Truth about Wheat, Carbs, and Sugars— Your Brain's Silent Killers.* Little, Brown and Company, New York, 2013.

56. Zeevi D, Korem T, Zmora N. Personalized nutrition by prediction of glycemic responses. *Cell* 2015;163(5):1079–94.

57. Korem T, Zeevi D, Zmora N et al. Bread affects clinical parameters and induces gut microbiome-associated personal glycemic responses. *Cell Metabolism* 2017;25(6):1243–53.

58. Biesiekierski JR, Peters SL, Newnham ED et al. No effects of gluten in patients with self-reported non-celiac gluten sensitivity after dietary reduction of fer-mentable, poorly absorbed, short-chain carbohydrates. *Gastroenterology* 2013;145(2):320–28.

59. Biesiekierski JR, Muir JG, Gibson PR. Is gluten a cause of gastrointestinal symp-toms in people without celiac disease? *Current Allergy and Asthma Reports* 2013;13(6):631–38.

60. Lebwohl B, Cao Y, Zong G. Long term gluten consumption in adults without celiac disease and risk of coronary heart disease: prospective cohort study. *BMJ* 2017;357.

61. Bulka CM, Davis MA. The unintended consequences of a gluten-free diet. *Epide-miology* 2017;28(3):24–25.

62. Dehghan M, Mente A, Zhang X et al. Associations of fats and carbohydrate intake with cardiovascular disease and mortality in 18 countries from five continents (PURE): a prospective cohort study. *Lancet* Epub ahead of print 2017; http://dx.doi .org/10.1016/S0140-6736(17)32252-3.

63. Ramsden CE, Domenichiello AF. PURE study challenges the definition of a healthy diet: but key questions remain. *Lancet* Epub ahead of print 2017; http:// dx.doi.org/10.1016/S0140-6736(17)32241-9.

# CHAPTER 7

1. Trumbo P, Schlicker S, Yates A A et al. Dietary reference intakes for energy, carbohydrates, fiber, fatty acids, cholesterol, protein, and amino acids. *Journal of the American Dietetic Association* 2002;102:1621–30.

2. Gortner WA. Nutrition in the United States: 1900-1974. *Cancer Research* 1975;35:3246–53.

3. Austin GL, Ogden OG, Hill JO. Trends in carbohydrate, fat, and protein intakes and association with energy intake in normal-weight, overweight, and obese individuals: 1971-2006. *American Journal of Clinical Nutrition* 2011;93(4):836–43.

4. Cordain L. *The Paleo Diet: Lose Weight and Get Healthy by Eating the Foods You Were Designed to Eat.* John Wiley and Sons, 2002.

5. Atkins R. *Dr. Atkins' Diet Revolution.* Random House, 1988.

6. Hartwig M. *The Whole30: The 30-Day Guide to Total Health and Food Freedom.* Houghton Mifflin Harcourt, 2015.

7. Westerterp KA. Diet-induced thermogenesis. *Nutrition & Metabolism* 2004;(1):5.

8. Pesta DH, Samuel VT. A high-protein diet for reducing body fat: mechanisms and possible caveats. *Nutrition & Metabolism* 2014;11:53–61.

9. Cuenca-Sanchez M, Navas-Carrillo D, Orenes-Pinero E. Controversies surrounding high-protein diet intake: satiating effect and kidney and bone health. *Advances in Nutrition* 2015;6:260–66.

10. Song M, Fung TT, Hu FB. Association of animal and plant protein intake with all-cause and cause-specific mortality. *JAMA Internal Medicine* 2016;176(10):1453–63.

11. Etemadi A, Sinha R, Ward MH et al. Mortality from different causes associated with meat, heme iron, nitrates, and nitrites in the NIH-AARP diet and health study: population based cohort study. *BMJ* 2017;357.

12. Hernandez-Alonso P, Salas-Salvado J, Ruiz-Canela M et al. High dietary protein intake is associated with an increased body weight and total death risk. *Clinical Nutrition* 2016;35(2):496–506.

13. Guevara-Aguirre J, Balasubramanian P, Guevara-Aguirre M et al. Growth hormone receptor deficiency is associated with major reduction in pro-aging signaling, cancer, and diabetes in humans. *Science Translational Medicine* 2011;3(70):70ra13.

14. Levine ME, Suarez JA, Brandhorst S et al. Low protein intake is associated with a major reduction in IGF-1, cancer, and overall mortality in the 65 and younger but not older population. *Cell Metabolism* 2014;19(3):407–17.

15. Stone TW, Darlington LG. Microbial carcinogenic toxins and dietary anti-cancer protectants. *Cellular and Molecular Life Sciences* 2017;74(14):2627–43.

16. Solon-Biet SM, McMahon AC, Ballard JW et al. The ratio of macronutrients, not caloric intake, dictates cardiometabolic health, aging, and longevity in ad libitum-fed mice. *Cell Metabolism* 2014;19(3):418–30.

## CHAPTER 8

1. http://www.vrg.org/nutshell/Polls/2016_adults_veg.htm
2. Asher K, Green C, Gutbrod H et al. Study of current and former vegetarians and vegans: initial study. Humane Resource Council, 2014, https://faunalytics.org/wp-content/uploads/2015/06/Faunalytics_Current-Former-Vegetarians_Full-Report.pdf.
3. Rosenfeld DL, Burrow AL. The unified model of vegetarian identity: A conceptual framework for understanding plant-based food choices. *Appetite* 2017;112(1):78–95.
4. Michalak J, Zhang XC, Jacobi F. Vegetarian diet and mental disorders: results from a representative community survey. *International Journal of Behavioral Nutrition and Physical Activity* 2012;9:67–81.
5. Bardone-Cone AM, Fitzsimmons-Craft EE, Harney MB et al. The interrelationships between vegetarianism and eating disorders among females. *Journal of the Academy of Nutrition and Dietetics* 2012;112(8):1247–52.
6. Zumonski K, Witte TK, Smith AR et al. Increased prevalence of vegetarianism among women with eating pathology. *Eating Behaviors* 2015;19:24–27.
7. Craig WJ. Health effects of vegan diets. *American Journal of Clinical Nutrition* 2009;89(5):16275–335.
8. Desai MS, Seekatz AM, Koropatkin NM et al. A dietary fiber-deprived gut microbiota degrades the colonic mucus barrier and enhances pathogen susceptibility. *Cell* 2016;167(5):1339–53.
9. Virtanen HEK, Kosikinen TT, Voutilainen S et al. Intake of different dietary proteins and risk of type 2 diabetes in men: the Kuopio ischaemic heart disease risk factor study. *British Journal of Nutrition* 2017;117(6):882–93.
10. Clarys P, Deliens T, Huybrechts I et al. Comparison of nutritional quality of the vegan, vegetarian, semi-vegetarian, pesco-vegetarian and omnivorous diet. *Nutrients* 2014;6(3):1318–32.
11. Dinu M, Abbate R, Gensini GF et al. Vegetarian, vegan diets and multiple health outcomes: a systematic review with meta-analysis of observational studies. *Critical Reviews in Food Science and Nutrition* 2017;57(17):3640–49.
12. Kahleova H, Klementova M, Herynek V et al. The effect of a vegetarian vs. conventional hypocaloric diabetic diet on thigh adipose tissue distribution in subjects

with type 2 diabetes: a randomized study. *Journal of the American College of Nutrition* 2017;36(5):364–69.

13. Kwok CS, Umar S, Myint PK et al. Vegetarian diet, Seventh Day Adventists and risk of cardiovascular mortality: a systematic review and meta-analysis. *International Journal of Cardiology* 2014:176(3):680–86.

14. Mihrshahi S, Ding D, Gale J et al. Vegetarian diet and all-cause mortality: evidence from a large population-based Australian cohort—the 45 and up study. *Preventive Medicine* 2017;97:1–7.

15. Satija A, Bhupathiraju SN, Spiegelman D et al. Healthful and unhealthful plant-based diets and the risk of coronary heart disease in US adults. *Journal of the American College of Cardiology* 2017;70(4):411–22.

16. Craig WJ. Health effects of vegan diets.

17. Louman MWJ, van Dusseldorp M, van de Vijver FJR et al. Signs of impaired cognitive function in adolescents with marginal cobalamin status. *American Journal of Clinical Nutrition* 2000;72(3):762–69.

18. Burke DG, Chilibeck PD, Parise G et al. Effect of creatine and weight training on muscle creatine and performance in vegetarians. *Medicine & Science in Sports & Exercise* 2003;35(11):1946–55.

19. Benton D, Donohoe R. The influence of creatine supplementation on the cognitive functioning of vegetarians and omnivores. *British Journal of Nutrition* 2011;105(7):1100–5.

20. Herrmann W, Schorr H, Obeid R et al. Vitamin B-12 status, particularly holotrans-cobalamin II and methylmalonic acid concentrations, and hyperhomocysteinemia in vegetarians. *American Journal of Clinical Nutrition* 2003;78(1):131–36.

21. Chiu YH, Afeiche MC, Williams PL et al. Fruit and vegetable intake and their pesticide residues in relation to semen quality among men from a fertility clinic. *Human Reproduction* 2015;30(6):1342–51.

22. Levine H, Swan S. Is dietary pesticide exposure related to semen quality? Positive evidence from men attending a fertility clinic. *Human Reproduction* 2015;30(6):1287–89.

23. https://www.ams.usda.gov/datasets/pdp

24. Kothapalli KSD, Ye K, Gadgil MS et al. Positive selection on a regulatory insertion-deletion polymorphism in FADS2 influences apparent endogenous synthesis of arachidonic acid. *Molecular Biology and Evolution* 2016;33(7):1726–39.

25. Stone TW, Darlington LG. Microbial carcinogenic toxins and dietary anti-cancer protectants. *Cellular and Molecular Life Sciences* 2017;74(14):2627–43.

26. Mahajani K, Bhatnagar V. Comparative study of prevalence of anaemia in vegetar-

ian and non-vegetarian woman of Udipaur City, Rajasthan. *Journal of Nutrition and Food Sciences* 2015;1–11.

27. Waldmann A, Koschizke JW, Leitzmann C et al. Dietary iron intake and iron status of German female vegans: results of the German vegan study. *Annals of Nutrition and Metabolism* 2004;48(2):103–8.

28. Hawk SN, Englehardt KG, Small C. Risks of iron deficiency among vegetarian college women. *Health* 2012;4(3):113–9.

29. Gonzalez R, Ballester I, Lopez-Posadas R et al. Effects of flavonoids and other polyphenols on inflammation. *Critical Reviews in Food Science and Nutrition* 2011;4(3):113–19.

30. Yang M, Lee G, Si J et al. Curcumin shows antiviral properties against norovirus. *Molecules* 2016;21:1401–15.

31. Kalashnikova I, Mazar J, Neal CJ et al. Nanoparticle delivery of curcumin induces cellular hypoxia and ROS-mediated apoptosis via modulation of Bcl-$_{2/B}$ax in human neuroblastoma. *Nanoscale* 2017;29:1–5.

32. Orzlowska E, Jacobson JJ, Bareh GM et al. Food intake diet and sperm characteristics in a blue zone: a Loma Linda Study. *European Journal of Obstetrics and Gynecology* 2016;5:43.

33. Bode A, Dong Z. Toxic phytochemicals and their potential risks for cancer. *Cancer Prevention Research* 2015;8(1):1–8.

34. Ghazarian H, Idoni B, Oppenheimer SB. A glycobiology review: carbohydrates, lectins and implications in cancer therapeutics. *Acta Histochemica* 2011;113:236–47.

35. Yue R, Shen B, Morrison SJ. Clec11a/osteolectin is an osteogenic growth factor that promotes the maintenance of the adult skeleton. *eLife* 2016;5:e18782.

36. Chan CKF, Ransom RC, Longaker MT. Lectins bring benefits to bones. *eLife* 2016;5:e22926.

37. Gundry SR. The Plant Paradox: The Hidden Dangers in "Healthy" Foods That Cause Disease and Weight Gain. Harper Wave, 2017.

38. Hamblin J. The next gluten. *The Atlantic* April 24, 2017, https://www.theatlantic.com/health/archive/2017/04/the-next-gluten/523686/.

39. Kreitman RJ. Taming ricin toxin. *Nature Biotechnology* 2003;21:372–74.

## CHAPTER 9

1. Halvorsen BL, Carlsen MH, Phillips KM et al. Content of redox-active compounds (i.e., antioxidants) in foods consumed in the United States. *American Journal of Clinical Nutrition* 2006;84(1):95–135.

2. Van Dam RM, Hu FB. Coffee consumption and risk of type 2 diabetes: a systematic review. *JAMA* 2005;294(1):97–104.

3. Ross GW, Abbott RD, Petrovitch H et al. Association of coffee and caffeine intake with the risk of Parkinson's disease. *JAMA* 2000;283:2674–79.

4. Saaksjarvi K, Knekt P, Rissanen H et al. Prospective study of coffee consumption and risk of Parkinson's disease. *European Journal of Clinical Nutrition* 2008;62:908–15.

5. Gardener H, Rundek T, Wright CB et al. Coffee and tea consumption are inversely associated with mortality in a multiethnic urban population. *Journal of Nutrition* 2013;143(8):1299–308.

6. Gunter MJ, Murphy N, Cross AJ et al. Coffee drinking and mortality in 10 European countries: a multinational cohort study. *Annals of Internal Medicine* 2017;July 11:1–26.

7. Park SY, Freedman ND, Haiman CA et al. Association of coffee consumption with total and cause-specific mortality among nonwhite populations. *Annals of Internal Medicine* 2017;167(4):228–35.

8. Ding M, Satija A, Bhupathiraju SN et al. Association of coffee consumption with total and cause-specific mortality in three large prospective cohorts. *Circulation* 2015;132(24):2305–15.

9. Arion WJ, Canfield WK, Ramos FC et al. Chlorogenic acid and hydronitrobenzaldehyde: New inhibitors of hepatic glucose 6-phosphatase. *Archives of Biochemistry and Biophysics* 1997;339:315–22.

10. Svilaas A, Sakhi AK, Andersen LF et al. Intakes of antioxidants in coffee, wine, and vegetables are correlated with plasma carotenoids in humans. *Journal of Nutrition* 2004;134:562–67.

11. McCusker RR, Fuerhrlein B, Goldberger BA et al. Caffeine content of decaffeinated coffee. *Journal of Analytical Toxicology* 2006;30:611–13.

12. Chen JF, Xu K, Petzer JP et al. Neuroprotection by caffeine and $A_{2A}$ adenosine receptor inactivation in a model of Parkinson's disease. *Journal of Neuroscience* 2001;21.

13. Furman D, Chang J, Lartigue L et al. Expression of specific inflammasome gene modules stratifies older individuals into two extreme clinical and immunological states. *Nature Medicine* 2017;23:174–84.

14. Captain Jean-Luc Picard (Patrick Stewart) in *Star Trek: The Next Generation*. Episode 211: "Contagion," 1989.

15. Tang J, Zheng JS, Fang L et al. Tea consumption and mortality of all cancers, CVD and all causes: a meta-analysis of eighteen prospective cohort studies. *British Journal of Nutrition* 2015;114(5):673-683.

16. Association of green tea consumption with mortality due to all causes and major causes of death in a Japanese Public Health Center-based Prospective Study (JPHC Study). *Annals of Epidemiology* 2015;25(7):512–18.

17. Feng L, Chong MS, Lim WS et al. Tea consumption reduces the incidence of neurocognitive disorders: finding from the Singapore Longitudinal Aging Study. *Journal of Nutrition, Health & Aging* 2016;20(10):1002–9.

18. Mandel SA, Kalfon AT, Reznichenko L et al. Targeting multiple neurodegenerative disease etiologies with multimodal-acting green tea catechins. *Journal of Nutrition* 2008;138:1578S–83S.

19. Tao L, Park JY, Lamber JD:. Differential prooxidative effects of the green tea polyphenol, (-)-epigallocatechin-3-gallate, in normal and oral cancer cells are related to differences in sirtulin 3 signaling. *Molecular Nutrition & Food Research* 2015;59(2):203–11.

20. Ek WE, Tobi EW, Ahsan M et al. Tea and coffee consumption in relation to DNA methylation in four European cohorts. *Human Molecular Genetics* 2017;26(16):3221–31.

21. Chang HC, Guarente L. SIRT1 mediates central circadian control in the SCN by a mechanism that decays with aging. *Cell* 2013;153(7):1448–60.

22. Lagouge M, Argmann C, Gerhart-Hines Z et al. Resveratrol improves mitochondrial function and protects against metabolic disease by activating SIRT1 and PGC-1alpha. *Cell* 2006;127(6):1109–22.

23. Chung S, Yao H, Caito S et al. Regulation of SIRT1 in cellular functions: role of polyphenols. *Archives of Biochemistry and Biophysics* 2010;501(1):79–90.

24. Asher G, Gatfield D, Stratmann M et al. SIRT1 regulates circadian clock gene expression through PER2 deacetylation. *Cell* 2008;134(2):317–28.

25. Nieves AR, Lucio M, Lima JL et al. Resveratrol in medicinal chemistry: a critical review of its pharmacokinetics, drug-delivery, and membrane interactions. *Current Medicinal Chemistry* 2012;19(11):1663–81.

26. Joseph JA, Fisher DR, Cheng V et al. Cellular and behavioral effects of stilbene resveratrol analogues; implications for reducing the deleterious effects of aging. *Journal of Agricultural and Food Chemistry* 2008;56(22):10544–51.

27. Pan Z, Agawal AK, Feng Q et al. Identification of molecular pathways affected by pterostilbene, a natural dimethylether analog of resveratrol. *BMC Medical Genomics* 2008;1–7.

28. Remsberg CM, Yanez JA, Ohgami Y et al. Pharmacometrics of pterostilbene: preclinical pharmacokinetics and metabolism, anticancer, anti-inflammatory, antioxidant and analgesic activity. *Phytotherapy Research* 2008;22(2):169–79.

29. Poulose SM, Thangthaeng N, Miller MG et al. Effects of pterostilbene and resveratrol on brain and behavior. *Neurochemistry International* 2015;89:227–33.
30. McCormack D, McFadden D. Pterostilbene and cancer: current review. *Journal of Surgical Research* 2012;173(2):53–61.
31. Kosuru R, Rai U, Prakash S et al. Promising therapeutic potential of pterostilbene and its mechanistic insight based on preclinical evidence. *European Journal of Pharmacology* 2016;789:229–43.
32. Wolf G. The discovery of the visual function of vitamin A. *Journal of Nutrition* 2001;131(6):1647–50.
33. Cabezas-Wallscheid N, Buettner F, Sommerkamp P et al. Vitamin A-retinoic acid signaling regulates hematopoietic stem cell dormancy. *Cell* 2017;169(5):807–23.
34. E. NAD+ in aging, metabolism, and neurodegeneration. *Science* 2015;350:1208–13. Imai S, Guarente L. NAD+ and sirtuins in aging and disease. *Trends in Cell Biology* 2014;24(8):464–71.
35. Chi Y, Sauve A. Nicotinamide riboside, a trace nutrient in foods, is a vitamin B$_3$ with effects on energy metabolism and neuroprotection. *Current Opinion in Clinical Nutrition and Metabolic Care* 2013;16(6):657–61.
36. Trammell SAJ, Schmidt MS, Weidemann BJ et al. Nicotinamide riboside is uniquely and orally bioavailable in mice and humans. *Nature Communications* 2016;4:1248–96.
37. Gong B, Pan Y, Vempati P et al. Nicotinamide riboside restores cognition through an upregulation of proliferator-activated receptor-gamma coactivator 1 alpha regulated beta-secretase 1 degradation and mitochondrial gene expression in Alzheimer's mouse models. *Neurobiology of Aging* 2013;34:1581–8.
38. Li J, Bonkowski MS, Moniot S et al. A conserved NAD+ binding pocket that regulates protein-protein interactions during aging. *Science* 2017;355(6331):1312–7.
39. Pauling L. *How to Live Longer and Feel Better*. WH Freedman, New York, 1986.
40. Hart A, Cota A, Makhdom A et al. The role of vitamin C in orthopedic trauma and bone health. *American Journal of Orthopedics* 2015;44(7):306–11.
41. Zollinger PE, Tuinebreijer WE, Kreis RW et al. Effect of vitamin C on frequency of reflex sympathetic dystrophy in wrist fractures: a randomized trial. *Lancet* 1999;11(354):2025–8.
42. Zollinger PE, Tuinebreijer WE, Breederveld, et al. Can vitamin C prevent complex regional pain syndrome in patients with wrist fractures? A randomized, controlled, multicenter dose-response study. *Journal of Bone and Joint Surgery. American Volume* 2007;89(7):1424–31.

43. Shibuya N, Humphers JM, Agarwal MR et al. Efficacy and safety of high-dose vitamin C on complex regional pain syndrome in extremity trauma and surgery—systematic review and meta-analysis. *Journal of Foot and Ankle Surgery* 2013;52:62–6.

44. Patton CM, Powell AP, Patel AA. Vitamin D in orthopaedics. *Journal of the American Academy of Orthopaedic Surgeons* 2012;20(3):123–9.

45. Angeline ME, Gee AO, Shindle M et al. The effects of vitamin D deficiency in athletes. *American Journal of Sports Medicine* 2013;41(2):461–4.

46. https://www.nasa.gov/feature/goddard/annual-antarctic-ozone-hole-larger-and -formed-later-in-2015

47. Patton CM. Vitamin D in orthopaedics. *JAAOS* 2012.

48. Narayanan DL, Saladi RN, Fox JL. Ultraviolet radiation and skin cancer. *International Journal of Dermatology* 210;49(9):978–86.

49. Brozyna A, Blazei Z, Ganese J et al. Mechanism of UV-related carcinogenesis and its contribution to nevi/melanoma. *Expert Review of Dermatology* 2007;2(4):451–69.

50. Chin K, Zhao D, Tibuakuu M et al. Physical activity, vitamin D, and incident atherosclerotic cardiovascular disease in whites and blacks: the ARIC study. *Journal of Clinical Endocrinology & Metabolism* 2017;102(4):1127–236.

51. Wright VJ. Osteoporosis in men. *Journal of the American Academy of Orthopaedic Surgeons* 2006;14(6):347–53.

52. Schnell S, Friedman SM, Mendelson DA et al. The 1-year mortality of patients treated in a hip fracture program for elders. *Geriatric Orthopaedic Surgery & Rehabilitation* 2010;1(1):6–14.

53. Fodor JG, Helis H, Yazdekhasti N et al. "Fishing" for the origins of "Eskimos and heart disease": facts or wishful thinking. *Canadian Journal of Cardiology* 2014;30(8):864–8.

54. Burr ML, Fehily AM, Gilbert JF et al. Effects of changes in fat, fish, and fibre intakes on death and myocardial reinfarction: diet and reinfarction trial (DART). *Lancet* 1989;2(8666):757–61.

55. Del Gobbo LC, Imamura F, Aslibekyan S et al. Omega-3 polyunsaturated fatty acid biomarkers and coronary heart disease: pooling project of 19 cohort studies. *JAMA Internal Medicine* 2016;176(8):1155–66.

56. Rizos EC, Ntzani EE, Bika E et al. Association between omega-3 fatty acid supplementation and risk of major cardiovascular disease events: a systematic review and meta-analysis. *JAMA* 2012;308(10):1024–33.

57. The Risk and Prevention Study Collaborative Group. N-3 fatty acids in patients with multiple cardiovascular risk factors. *New England Journal of Medicine* 2013;368:1800–8.

58. Grey A, Bollard M. Clinical trial evidence and use of fish oil supplements. *JAMA Internal Medicine* 2014;174(3):460–2.

59. Mason RR, Sherratt SC. Omega-3 fatty acid fish oil dietary supplements contain saturated fats and oxidized lipids that may interfere with their intended biological benefits. *Biochemical and Biophysical Research Communications* 2017;483(1):425–9.

60. Fialkow J. Omega-3 fatty acid formulations in cardiovascular disease: dietary supplements are not substitutes for prescription products. *American Journal of Cardiovascular Drugs* 2016;16:229–39.

61. Brasky TM, Darke AK, Song X et al. Plasma phospholipid fatty acids and prostate cancer risk in the SELECT trial. *Journal of the National Cancer Institute* 2013;105(15):1132–41.

# CHAPTER 10

1. Lewis GD, Farrell L, Wood MJ et al. Metabolic signatures of exercise in human plasma. *Science Translational Medicine* 2010;2(33):33–7.

2. Mattheson GO, Klugl M, Engebretsen L et al. Prevention and management of non-communicable disease: the IOC consensus statement, Lausanne 2013. *Sports Medicine* 2013;43(11):1075–88.

3. Lavie CJ, Lee DC, Sui X. Effects of running on chronic diseases and cardiovascular and all-cause mortality. *Mayo Clinic Proceedings* 2015;90(11):1541–52.

4. Lee DC, Pate RR, Lavie CJ et al. Leisure-time running reduces all-cause and cardiovascular mortality risk. *Journal of the American College of Cardiology* 204;64(5):472–81.

5. Northey JM, Cherbuin NM, Pumpa KL et al. Exercise interventions for cognitive function in adults older than 50: a systematic review with meta-analysis. *British Journal of Sports Medicine* 2016:096587.

6. Dolezal BA, Neufeld EV, Boland DM et al. Interrelationship between sleep and exercise: a systematic review. *Advances in Preventive Medicine* 2017;1364387.

7. Gillen JB, Martin BJ, MacInnis MJ et al. Twelve weeks of sprint interval training improves indices of cardiometabolic health similar to traditional endurance training despite a five-fold lower exercise volume and time commitment. *PLOS One* 2016;11(4):e0154075.

8. Overgaard M, Rasmussen P, Bohm AM et al. Hypoxia and exercise provoke both lactate release and lactate oxidation by the human brain. *FASEB Journal* 2012;26(7):3012–20.

9. Teschendorff AE, West J, Beck S. Age-associated epigenetic drift: implications, and a case of epigenetic thrift? *Human Molecular Genetics* 2013;22:r7–r15.

10. Barres R, Yan J, Egan B et al. Acute exercise remodels promoter methylation in human skeletal muscle. *Cell Metabolism* 2012;15:405–11.

11. Lindholm ME, Marabita F, Gomez-Cabrero D et al. An integrative analysis reveals coordinated reprogramming of the epigenome and the transcriptome in human skeletal muscle after training. *Epigenetics* 2014;9(12):1557–69.

12. Cherkas LF, Hunkin JL, Kato BS et al. The association between physical activity in leisure time and leukocyte telomere length. *Archives of Internal Medicine* 2008;168(2):154–8.

13. Werner C, Furster T, Widmann T et al. Physical exercise prevents cellular senescence in circulating leukocytes and in the vessel wall. *Circulation* 2009;120(24):2438–47.

14. Tucker LA. Physical activity and telomere length in US men and women: an NHANES investigation. *Preventive Medicine* 2017;100:145–51.

15. Diman A, Boros J, Poulain F et al. Nuclear respiratory factor 1 and endurance exercise promote human telomerase transcription. *Science Advances* 2016;2(7):e1600031.

16. Philip A, Schenk S. Unraveling the complexities of SIRT1-mediated mitochondrial regulation in skeletal muscle. *Exercise and Sport Sciences Reviews* 2013;41(3):174–81.

17. Sahin E, Colla S, Liesa M et al. Telomere dysfunction induces metabolic and mitochondrial compromise. *Nature* 2011;470:359–65.

18. Overmyer KA, Evans CR, Qi NR et al. Maximal oxidative capacity during exercise is associated with skeletal muscle fuel selection and dynamic changes in mitochondrial protein acetylation. *Cell Metabolism* 2015;21(3):468–78.

19. Safdar A, Bourgeois JM, Ogborn DI et al. Endurance exercise rescues progeroid aging and induces systemic mitochondrial rejuvenation in mitochondrial DNA mutator mice. *PNAS* 2011;108(10):4135–40.

20. Clark-Matott J, Saleem A, Dai Y et al. Metabolomic analysis of exercise effects in the POLG mitochondrial DNA mutator mouse brain. *Neurobiology of Aging* 2015;36(11):2972–83.

21. Blumenthal JA, Babyak MA, Moore KA et al. Effects of exercise training on older patients with major depression. *Archives of Internal Medicine* 1999;159(19):2349–56.

22. McGarrah RW, Slentz CA, Kraus WE. The effect of vigorous- versus moderate-intensity aerobic exercise on insulin action. *Current Cardiology Reports* 2016;18(12):117.
23. Neufer PO, Bamman MM, Muoio DM et al. Understanding the cellular and molecular mechanisms of physical activity-induced health benefits. *Cell Metabolism* 2015;22(1):4–11.
24. Xu B. BDNF rising from exercise. *Cell Metabolism* 2013;18(5):612–4.
25. Wrann CD, White JP, Salogiannnis J et al. Exercise induces hippocampal BDNF through a PGC-1 alpha/FNDC5 pathway. *Cell Metabolism* 2013;18(5):649–59.
26. Takinmoto M, Hamada T. Acute exercise increases brain region-specific expression of MCT1, MCT2, MCT4, GLUT1, and COX IV proteins. *Journal of Applied Physiology* 2014;116(9):1238–50.
27. Naci H, Ioannidis JPA. Comparative effectiveness of exercise and drug interventions on mortality outcomes: metaepidemiological study. *BMJ* 2013;347:f5577.
28. Raichlen DA, Alexander GE. Adaptive capacity: an evolutionary neuroscience model linking exercise, cognition, and brain health. *Trends in Neuroscience* 2017;40(7):408–21.
29. Kjolhede T, Siemonsen S, Wenzel D et al. Can resistance training impact MRI outcomes in relapse-remitting multiple sclerosis? *Multiple Sclerosis Journal* 2017;21(5):599–611.
30. Jenkins NDM, Miramonti AA, Hill EC et al. Greater neural adaptations following high- vs. low-load resistance training. *Frontiers in Physiology* 2017;8:331.

## CHAPTER 11

1. Melov S, Tarnopolsky MA, Hubbard A, et al. Resistance exercise reverses aging in human skeletal muscle. *PLOS One* 2007;2(5):e465.
2. Zykovich A, Hubbard A, Flynn JM et al. Genome-wide DNA methylation changes with age in disease-free human skeletal muscle. *Aging Cell* 2014;13(2):360–6.
3. Denham J, Marques FZ, Bruns EL et al. Epigenetic changes in leucocytes after 8 weeks of resistance exercise training. *European Journal of Applied* Moore SC, Patel AV, Matthews CE et al. Leisure time physical activity of moderate to vigorous intensity and mortality: a large pooled cohort analysis. *PLOS Medicine* 2012;9(11):e1001335.
4. Buckner SL, Dankel SJ, Mattocks KT et al. The problem of muscle hypertrophy: revisited. *Muscle & Nerve* 2016;54(6):1012–14.
5. Timmins KA, Leech RD, Batt ME et al. Running and knee osteoarthritis: a systematic review and meta-analysis. *American Journal of Sports Medicine* 2017;45(6):1447–57.

6. Lavie CJ, Lee DC, Sui X. Effects of running on chronic diseases and cardiovascular and all-cause mortality. *Mayo Clinic Proceedings* 2015;90(11):1541–52.
7. Oja P, Kelly P, Titze S et al. Associations of specific types of sports and exercise with all-cause and cardiovascular-disease mortality: a cohort study of 80,306 British adults. *British Journal of Sports Medicine* 2017;51(10):812–17.
8. Lee DC, Brellenthin AG, Thompson PD et al. Running as a key lifestyle medicine for longevity. *Progress in Cardiovascular Diseases* 2017;60(1):45–55.
9. Lee DC, Pate RR, Lavie CJ et al. Leisure-time running reduces all-cause and cardiovascular mortality risk. *Journal of the American College of Cardiology* 2014;64(5):472–81.
10. Hsu CL, Best JR, Davis JC et al. Aerobic exercise promotes executive functions and impacts functional neural activity among older adults with vascular cognitive impairment. *British Journal of Sports Medicine* 2017;0:19.
11. Thomas RJ, Kenfield SA, Jimenez JA: Exercise-induced biochemical changes and their potential influence on cancer. Br J Sports Med 2017;51:640-644.
12. Baipeyi S, Covington JD, Taylor EM et al. Skeletal muscle PGC1-alpha -1 nucleosome position and -260 nt DNA methylation determine exercise response and prevent ectopic lipid accumulation in men. *Endocrinology* 2017;158(7):2190–9.
13. Pedersen L, Idorn M, Olofsson GH et al. Voluntary running suppresses tumor growth through epinephrine- and IL-6-dependent NK cell mobilization and redistribution. *Cell Metabolism* 2016;23(3):554–62.
14. Ornish D, Lin J, Chan JM et al. Effect of comprehensive lifestyle changes on telomerase activity and telomeric length in men with biopsy-proven low-risk prostate cancer: 5-year follow-up of a descriptive pilot study. *Lancet Oncology* 2013;14(11):1112–20.
15. Ntanasis-Stathopoulos J, Tzanninis J, Philippou A et al. Epigenetic regulation on gene expression induced by physical exercise. *Journal of Musculoskeletal & Neuronal Interactions* 2013;13(2):133–46.
16. Chin K, Zhao D, Tibuakuu M et al. Physical activity, vitamin D, and incident atherosclerotic cardiovascular disease in whites and blacks: the ARIC study. *Journal of Clinical Endocrinology and Metabolism* 2017;102(4):1227–236.
17. Silvennoinen M, Ahtiainen JP, Hulmi JJ et al. PGC-1 alpha isoforms and their target genes are expressed differently in human skeletal muscle following resistance and endurance exercise. *Physiological Reports* 2015;3:e12563.
18. Davy BM, Winett RA, Savia J et al. Resist diabetes: a randomized clinical trial for resistance training maintenance in adults with prediabetes. *PLOS One* 2017;0172610.

19. Volaklis KA, Halle M, Meisinger C. Muscular strength as a strong predictor of mortality: a narrative review. *European Journal of Internal Medicine* 2015;26(5):303–10.

20. Cooper R, Kuh D, Hardy R et al. Objectively measured physical capability levels and mortality: systematic review and meta-analysis. *BMJ* 2010;341:c4467.

21. Ruiz JR, Sui X, Lobelo F et al. Association between muscular strength and mortality in men: prospective cohort study. *BMJ* 2008;337(7661):92–5.

22. Kraschnewski JL, Sciamanna CN, Poger JM et al. Is strength training associated with mortality benefits? A 15-year cohort study of US older adults. *Preventive Medicine* 2016;87:121–7.

23. Daabis R, Hassan M, Zidan M. Endurance and strength training in pulmonary rehabilitation for COPD patients. *Egyptian Journal of Chest Disease and Tuberculosis* 2017;66(2):231–66.

24. Krist L, Dimeo F, Keil T. Can progressive resistance training twice a week improve mobility, muscle strength, and quality of life in very elderly nursing-home residents with impaired mobility? A pilot study. *Clinical Interventions in Aging* 2013;8:443–8.

25. Steele J, Raubold K, Kemmler W et al. The effects of 6 months of progressive high effort resistance training methods upon strength, body composition, function, and wellbeing of elderly adults. *BioMed Research International* 2017;(2017):1–14, article ID 2541090.

26. Merkary RA, Grontved A, Despres JP et al. Weight training, aerobic physical activities, and long-term waist circumference change in men. *Obesity* 2015;23(2):461–7.

27. Howe TE, Shea B, Dawson LJ et al. Exercise for preventing and treating osteoporosis in postmenopausal women. *Cochrane Database of Systematic Reviews* 2011:6(7):CD000333.

28. Tai V, Leung W, Grey A et al. Calcium intake and bone mineral density: systematic review and meta-analysis. *BMJ* 2015;351:h4183.

29. Melov S, Tarnoppolsky MA, Beckman K et al. Resistance exercise reverses aging in *Physiology* 2016;116(6):1245–53.

30. Rea IM. Towards ageing well: use it or lose it: exercise, epigenetics and cognition. *Biogerontology* 2017;18(4):679–91.

31. Loehr JA, Lee SMC, English KL et al. Musculoskeletal adaptations to training with the Advanced Resistive Training Device. *Medicine & Science in Sports & Exercise* 2011;43(1):146–56.

32. Meyer J, Morrison J, Zuniga J. The benefits and risks of CrossFit: a systematic review. *Workplace Health Safety* 2017;2165079916685568.

33. Kliszczewicz B, Quindry CJ, Blessing LD et al. Acute exercise and oxidative stress: CrossFit vs treadmill bout. *Journal of Human Kinetics* 2015;14(47):81–90.

34. Metcalfe RS, Babtaj JA, Fawkner SG et al. Towards the minimal amount of exercise for improving metabolic health: beneficial effects of reduced-exertion high-intensity interval training. *European Journal of Applied Physiology* 2012;112(7):2767–75.

35. Weston KS, Wisloff U, Coombes JS. High-intensity interval training in patients with lifestyle-induced cardiometabolic disease: a systematic review and meta-analysis. *British Journal of Sports Medicine* 2014;48(16):1227–34.

36. Rognmo O, Moholdt T, Baaken H et al. Cardiovascular risk of high- versus moderate-intensity aerobic exercise in coronary heart disease patients. *Circulation* 2012;126(12):1436–40.

37. Boutcher S. High-intensity intermittent exercise and fat loss. *Journal of Obesity* 2011;868305.

38. Trapp EG, Chisholm DJ, Freund J. The effects of high-intensity intermittent exercise training on fat loss and fasting insulin levels of young women. *International Journal of Obesity* 2008;32(4):684–91.

39. Smith MM, Sommer AJ, Starkoff BE. CrossFit-based high-intensity power training improves maximal aerobic fitness and body composition. *Journal of Strength & Conditioning Research* 2013;27(11):3159–72.

40. Robinson MM, Dasari S, Konopka AR et al. Enhanced protein translation underlies improved metabolic and physical adaptations to different exercise training modes in young and old humans. *Cell Metabolism* 2017;25(3):581–92.

41. Klimek C, Ashbeck C, Brook AJ et al. Are injuries more common with CrossFit training than other forms of exercise? *Journal of Sport Rehabilitation* 2017;2:1–17.

42. Moran S, Booker H, Staines J et al. Rates and risk factors of injury in CrossFit: a prospective cohort study. *Journal of Sports Medicine and Physical Fitness* 2017;57(9):1147–53.

43. Weisenthal BM, Beck CA, Maloney MD et al. Injury rate and patterns among CrossFit athletes. *Orthopaedic Journal of Sports Medicine* 2014;2(4):2325967114531177.

44. Arem H, Moore SC, Patel A et al. Leisure time activity and mortality: a detailed pooled analysis of the dose-response relationship. *JAMA Internal Medicine* 2015;175(6):959–67.

45. Gillen JB, Martin BJ, MacInnis MJ et al. Twelve weeks of sprint interval training improves indices of cardiometabolic health similar to traditional endurance training despite a five-fold lower exercise volume and time commitment. *PLOS One* 2016;11(4):e0154075.

# CHAPTER 12

1. Curlik DM, Maeng LY, Agarwal PR et al. Physical skill training increases the number of surviving new cells in the adult hippocampus. *PLOS One* 2013;8:e55850.

2. Van Praag H, Kempermann G, Gage RH et al. Running increases cell proliferation and neurogenesis in the adult mouse dentate gyrus. *Nature Neuroscience* 19992:2666-270.

3. Eisch AJ, Petrik D. Depression and hippocampal neurogenesis: a road to remission? *Science* 2012;338(6103):72–5.

4. Buric I, Farias M, Jong J et al. What is the molecular signature of mind-body interventions? A systematic review of gene expression changes induced by meditation and related practices. *Frontiers in Immunology* 2017;8:670.

5. Alderman BL, Olson RL, Brush CJ et al. MAP training: combining meditation and aerobic exercise reduces depression and rumination while enhancing synchronized brain activity. *Translational Psychology* 2016;6:e726.

6. Buric et al. Gene expression induced by meditation. *Frontiers in Immunology* 2017 (see reference #4).

7. Dusek JA, Otu HH, Wohlhueter AL et al. Genomic counter-stress changes induced by the relaxation response. *PLOS One* 2008;3(7):e2576.

8. Bhasin MK, Dusek JA, Chang B-H et al. Relaxation response induces temporal transcriptome changes in energy metabolism, insulin secretion, and inflammatory pathways. *PLOS One* 2013;8(5):e62817.

9. Benson H, Beary JF, Carol MP. The relaxation response. *Psychiatry* 1974;37(1):37-46.

10. Carlson LE, Beattie TL, Giese-Davis J, et al. Mindfulness-based cancer recovery and supportive-expressive therapy maintain telomere length relative to controls in distressed breast cancer survivors. *Cancer* 2015;121(3):476–84.

11. Ravnik-Glavac M, Hrašovec S, Bon J et al. Genome-wide expression changes in a higher state of consciousness. *Consciousness and Cognition* 2012;21(3):1322–44.

12. Chu P, Gotink RA, Yeh GY. The effectiveness of yoga in modifying risk factors for cardiovascular disease and metabolic syndrome: a systematic review and meta-analysis of randomized controlled trials. *European Journal of Preventive Cardiology* 2016;3(3):291–307.

13. Field T. Yoga clinical research review. *Complementary Therapies in Clinical Practice* 2011;17(1):1–8.

14. Kristal AR, Littman AJ, Benitez D et al. Yoga practice is associated with attenuated weight gain in healthy, middle-aged men and women. *Alternative Therapies in Health and Medicine* 2005;11(4):28–33.

15. Hagins M, States R, Selfe T et al. Effectiveness of yoga for hypertension: systematic review and meta-analysis. *Evidence-Based Complementary and Alternative Medicine* 2013;e649836:1–13.

16. Uebelacker LA, Tremont G, Gillette LT et al. Adjunctive yoga v. health education for persistent major depression: a randomized controlled trial. *Psychological Medicine* 2017;47(12):2130–42.

17. Ben-Josef AM, Chen J, Wileto P et al. Effect of Eischens yoga during radiation therapy on prostate cancer patient symptoms and quality of life: a randomized phase II trial. *International Journal of Radiation Oncology, Biology, Physics* 2017;98(5):1036–44.

18. Tilbrook HE, Cox H, Hewitt CE et al. Yoga for chronic low back pain. *Annals of Internal Medicine* 2011;155(9):569–78.

19. Hagins M, States R, Selfe T et al. Effectiveness of yoga for hypertension: systematic review and meta-analysis. *Evidence-Based Complementary and Alternative Medicine* 2013;e649836:1–13.

20. Holtzman S, Beggs RT. Yoga for chronic low back pain: a meta-analysis of randomized controlled trials. *Pain Research & Management* 2013;18(5):267–72.

21. Saper RNB, Lemaster C, Delitto A et al. Yoga, physical therapy, or education for chronic lower back pain: a randomized noninferiority trial. *Annals of Internal Medicine* 2017;167(2):85–94.

22. Groessi EJ, Liu L, Chang DG et al. Yoga for military veterans with chronic low back pain: a randomized clinical trial. *American Journal of Preventive Medicine* July 2017, epub ahead of press.

23. Eyre HA, Acevedo B, Yang H. Changes in neural connectivity and memory following yoga intervention for older adults: a pilot study. *Journal of Alzheimer's Disease* 2016;52(2):673–85.

24. Harkess KN, Ryan J, Delfabbro PH et al. Preliminary indications of the effect of a brief yoga intervention on markers of inflammation and DNA methylation in chronically stressed women. *Translational Psychiatry* 2016;6:e965.

25. Campo M, Shiyo MP, Kean MB et al. Musculoskeletal pain associated with recreational yoga participation: a prospective cohort study with 1-year follow-up. *Journal of Bodywork and Movement Therapies* 2017; article in press.

26. Wang N, Zhang X, Xiang YB et al. Associations of walking, jogging, and tai chi with mortality in Chinese men. *American Journal of Epidemiology* 2013;178(5):791–6.

27. Song R, Lee EO, Lam P et al. Effects of tai chi exercise on pain, balance, muscle strength, and perceived difficulties in physical function in older women with osteoarthritis: a randomized clinical trial. *Journal of Rheumatology* 2003:30(9):2039–44.

28. Lomas-Vega R, Obrero-Gaitán E, Molina-Ortega FJ et al. Tai chi for risk of falls. A meta-analysis. *Journal of the American Geriatrics Society* 2017;doi:10.1111 /jgs.15008, epub ahead of print.

29. Yeung AS, Feng R, Hyung Kim DJ et al. A pilot, randomized controlled study of tai chi with passive and active controls in the treatment of depressed Chinese-Americans. *Journal of Clinical Psychiatry* 2017;78(5):e522–8.

30. Chen YW, Hunt MA, Campbell KL et al. The effect of tai chi on four chronic conditions—cancer, osteoarthritis, heart failure and chronic obstructive pulmonary disease: a systematic review and meta-analyses. *British Journal of Sports Medicine* 2016:50(7):397–424.

31. Shi ZM, Wen HP, Liu FR et al. The effects of tai chi on the renal and cardiac functions of patients with chronic kidney and cardiovascular diseases. *Journal of Physical Therapy Science* 2014;26(11):1733–6.

32. Lauche R, Stumpe C, Fehr J et al. The effects of tai chi and neck exercises in the treatment of chronic nonspecific neck pain: a randomized controlled trial. *Journal of Pain* 2016;17(9):1013–27.

33. Taggart HM, Arslanian CL, Bae S et al. Effects of t'ai chi exercise on fibromyalgia symptoms and health-related quality of life. *Orthopedic Nursing* 2003;22(5):353–60.

34. Wang C, Schmid CH, Rones R et al. A randomized trial of tai chi for fibromyalgia. *New England Journal of Medicine* 2010;363:743–54.

35. Goon JA, Noor Aini AH, Musalmah M et al. Effect of tai chi exercise on DNA damage, antioxidant enzymes, and oxidative stress in middle-age adults. *Journal of Human Kinetics* 2009:6(1):43–54.

36. Ren H, Collins V, Clarke SJ et al. Epigenetic changes in response to tai chi practice: a pilot investigation of DNA methylation marks. *Evidence-Based Complementary and Alternative Medicine* 2012;e841810:1–9.

37. Segal N, Hein J, Basford JR. The effects of Pilates training on flexibility and body composition: an observational study. *Archives of Physical Medicine and Rehabilitation* 2004;85(12):1977–81.

38. Newell D, Shead V, Sloane L. Changes in gait and balance parameters in elderly subjects attending an 8-week supervised Pilates programme. *Journal of Bodywork and Movement Therapies* 2012;16(4):549–54.

39. Bird ML, Fell J. Positive long-term effects of Pilates exercise on the aged-related decline in balance and strength in older, community-dwelling men and women. *Journal of Aging and Physical Activity* 2016;22(3):342–7.

40. Fox EE, Hough AD, Creanor S et al. Effects of Pilates-based core stability training in ambulant people with multiple sclerosis: multicenter, assessor-blinded, randomized controlled trial. *Physical Therapy* 2016;96(8):1170–8.

## CHAPTER 13

1. Krause N. Meaning in life and mortality. *Journals of Gerontology Series B: Psychological Sciences and Social Sciences* 2009;64B(4):517–27. Hill PL, Turiano NA. Purpose in life as a predictor of mortality across adulthood. *Psychological Science* 2014;25(7):1482–6.

2. Levy BR, Slade MD, Kunkel SR et al. Longevity increased by positive self-perceptions of aging. *Journal of Personality and Social Psychology* 2002;83(2):261–70.

3. Boyle PA, Barnes LL, Buchman AS et al. Purpose in life is associated with mortality among community-dwelling older persons. *Psychosomatic Medicine* 2009;71(5):574–9.

4. Cohen R, Chirag B, Rozanski A. Purpose in life and its relationship to all-cause mortality and cardiovascular events: a meta-analysis. *Psychosomatic Medicine* 2016;78(2):122–33.

5. Koizumi M, Ito H, Kaneko Y et al. Effect of having a sense of purpose in life on the risk of death from cardiovascular diseases. *Journal of Epidemiology* 2008;18(5):191–6.

6. Yu L, Boyle PA, Wilson RS et al. Purpose in life and cerebral infarcts in community-dwelling older people. *Stroke* 2015;46(4):1071–6.

7. Levy BR, Slade MD, Murphy TE et al. Association between positive age stereotypes and recovery from disability in older persons. *JAMA* 2012;308(19):1972–3.

8. Boyle PA, Buchman AS, Bennett DA. Purpose in life is associated with a reduced risk of incident disability among community-dwelling older persons. *American Journal of Geriatric Psychology* 2010;18(12):1093–102.

9. Levy BR, Ferrucci L, Zonderman AB et al. A culture-brain link: negative age stereotypes predict Alzheimer's disease biomarkers. *Psychology and Aging* 2016;31(1):82–8.

10. Boyle PA, Buchman AS, Wilson RS et al. Effect of purpose in life on the relation between Alzheimer disease pathologic changes on cognitive function in advanced age. *Archives of General Psychiatry* 2012;69(5):499–505.

11. Hill PL, Turiano NA, Mroczek DK et al. The value of a purposeful life: sense of value predicts greater income and net worth. *Journal of Research in Personality* 2016;65:38–42.

12. Zaninotto P, Wardle J, Steptoe A. Sustained enjoyment of life and mortality at older ages: analysis of the English Longitudinal Study of Ageing. *BMJ* 2016;355:i6267.

13. KC and the Sunshine Band: *Get Down Tonight,* 1975; Harry Wayne Casey and Richard Finch.

14. Rebok GW, Ball K, Guey LT et al. Ten-year effects of the ACTIVE cognitive training trial on cognition and everyday functioning in older adults. *Journal of the American Geriatrics Society* 2014;62(1):16–24.

15. https://www.brainhq.com/why-brainhq

16. Smith GE, Housen P, Yaffe K et al. A cognitive training program based on principles on brain plasticity: results from the Improvement in Memory with Plasticity-based Adaptive Cognitive Training (IMPACT) study. *Journal of the American Geriatrics Society* 2009;57(4):594–603.

17. Anguera JA, Boccanfuso J, Rintoul JL et al. Video game training enhances cognitive control in older adults. *Nature* 2013;501(7465):97–101.

18. Melby-Lervag M, Hulme C. Is working memory training effective? A meta-analytic review. *Developmental Psychology* 2013;49(2):270–91.

19. Simon DJ, Boot WR, Charness N et al. Do "brain training" programs work? *Psychological Science in the Public Interest* 2016;17(3):103–86.

20. Kim S, Hasher L, Zacks RT. Aging and a benefit of distractibility. *Psychonomic Bulletin & Review* 2007;14(2):301–5.

21. Campbell KL, Hasher L, Thomas RC. Hyper-binding: a unique age effect. *Psychological Science* 2010;2(3):399–405.

22. Carsen SH, Peterson JB, Higgins DM. Decreased latent inhibition is associated with increased creative achievement in high-functioning individuals. *Journal of Personality and Social Psychology* 2003;85(3):499–506.

23. Ansburg PI, Hill K. Creative and analytic thinkers differ in their use of attentional resources. *Personality and Individual Differences* 2003;34(7):1141–52.

24. Salat DH, Buckner RL, Snyder AZ et al. Thinning of the cerebral cortex in aging. *Cerebral Cortex* 2004;14(1):721–30.

25. Dotson VM, Szymkowicz SM, Sozda CN et al. Age differences in prefrontal sur-face area and thickness in middle aged to older adults. *Frontiers in Aging Neuro-science* 2016;7:250.

26. Csikszentmihalyi M. Flow: *The Psychology of Optimal Experience*. Harper and Row, 1990.

27. Miranda RA, Casebeer WA, Hein AM et al. DARPA-funded efforts in the devel-opment of novel brain-computer interface technologies. *Journal of Neuroscience Methods* 2015;244(4):52–67.

28. Kotler S. *The Rise of Superman*. Houghton, Mifflin, Harcourt, 2014.

29. Beckes L, Coan JA, Hasselmo K. Familiarity promotes the blurring of self and other in the neural representation of threat. *Social Cognitive and Affective Neuro-science* 2012;8(6):670–7.

30. Rizzolatti G, Craighero L. The mirror neuron system. *Annual Review of Neurosci-ence* 2004;27(1):169–92.

## CHAPTER 14

1. Travison TG, Araujo AB, O'Donnell AB et al. A population-level decline in serum testosterone levels in American men. *Journal of Clinical Endocrinology and Metab-olism* 2007;92(1):196–202.

2. Bhasin S. Secular decline in male reproductive function: is manliness threatened? *Journal of Clinical Endocrinology and Metabolism* 2007;92(1):44–5.

3. Bermon S, Garnier PY. Serum androgen levels and their relation to performance in track and field: mass spectrometry results from 2127 observations in male and female elite athletes. *British Journal of Sports Medicine* 2017:e097792.

4. Baillargeon J, Urban RJ, Ottenbacher KJ et al. Trends in androgen prescribing in the United States, 2001-2011. *JAMA Internal Medicine* 2013;173(15):1465–6.

5. Lukyanenko YO, Chen JJ, Hutson JC. Production of 25-hydroxycholesterol by tes-ticular macrophages and its effects on Leydig cells. *Biology of Reproduction* 2001;64(3):790–6.

6. Duan L, Zhu J, Wang K et al. Does fluoride affect serum testosterone and andro-gen binding with age-specificity? A population-based cross-sectional study in Chinese male farmers. *Biological Trace Element Research* 2016;174(2):294–9.

7. Pitz S, Frisch S, Koertke H et al. Effect of vitamin D supplementation on testoster-one levels in men. *Hormone and Metabolic Research* 2011:43(3):223–5.

8. Wu FC, Tajar A, Beynon JM et al. Identification of late-onset hypogonadism in middle-aged and elderly men. *New England Journal of Medicine* 2010;363:123–35.

9. Ramasamy R, Golan R, Wilken N et al. Association of free testosterone with hypo-gonadal symptoms in men with near-normal total testosterone levels. *Urology* 2015;86(2):287–90.

10. Harman SM, Metter EJ, Tobin JD et al. Longitudinal effects of aging on serum total and free testosterone levels in healthy men. Baltimore Longitudinal Study of Aging. *Journal of Clinical Endocrinology and Metabolism* 2001;86(2):724–31.

11. Cheetham TC, An JJ, Jacobsen SJ et al. Association of testosterone replacement with cardiovascular outcomes among men with androgen deficiency *JAMA Internal Medicine* 2017;177(4):491–9.

12. Muraleedharan V, Marsh H, Kapoor D et al. Testosterone deficiency is associated with increased risk of mortality and testosterone replacement improves survival in men with type 2 diabetes. *European Journal of Endocrinology* 2013;169(6):725–33.

13. Jones TH, Arver S, Behre HM et al. Testosterone replacement in hypogonadal men with type 2 diabetes and/or metabolic syndrome (the TIMES2 study). *Diabetes Care* 2011;34(4):828–37.

14. Snyder PJ, Bhasin S, Cunningham GR et al. Effects of testosterone treatment in older men. *New England Journal of Medicine* 2016;374:611–24.

15. Orwoll ES. Establishing a framework—does testosterone supplementation help older men? *New England Journal of Medicine* 2016;374:682–3.

16. Spitzer M, Basaria S, Travison TG et al. Effect of testosterone replacement on response to sildenafil citrate in men with erectile dysfunction: a parallel, random-ized trial. *Annals of Internal Medicine* 2012;157(10):681–91.

17. Isodori AM, Giannetta E, Gianfrilli D et al. Effects of testosterone on sexual func-tion in men: results of a meta-analysis. *Clinical Endocrinology* 2005;63(4):381–4.

18. Cororna G, Sforza A, Maggi M. Testosterone replacement therapy: long-term safety and efficacy. *World Journal of Men's Health* 2017; in press.

19. Basaria S, Coviello AD, Travison TG et al. Adverse events associated with testos-terone administration. *New England Journal of Medicine* 2010;363:109–22.

20. Bhasin S, Cunningham GR, Hayes FJ et al. Testosterone therapy in men with androgen deficiency syndromes: an Endocrine Society clinical practice guideline. *Journal of Clinical Endocrinology and Metabolism* 2010;95(6):2536–59.

21. Mueleman EJH, Legros J, Bouloux PMG et al. Effects of long-term oral testosterone undecanoate therapy on urinary symptoms: data from a 1-year, placebo-controlled, dose-ranging trial in aging men with symptomatic hypogonadism. *Aging Male* 2015;18(3):157–63.

22. Corona G, Rastrelli G, Morgentaler A et al. Meta-analysis of results of testosterone therapy on sexual function based on international index of erectile function scores. *European Urology* 2017; in press.

23. Mehtal PH, Beer J. Neural mechanisms of the testosterone-aggression relation: the role of orbitofrontal cortex. *Journal of Cognitive Neuroscience* 2010;22(10):2357–68.

24. Nave G, Nadler A, Zava D et al. Single-dose testosterone administration impairs cognitive reflection in men. *Psychological Science* 2017; in press.

25. Wright ND, Bahrami B, Johnson E et al. Testosterone disrupts human collaboration by increasing egocentric choices. *Proceedings. Biological Sciences* 2012;279(1736):2275–80.

26. Walters MJ. The growth hormone receptor. *Growth Hormone & IGF Research* 2016;28:6–10.

27. Rudman D, Feller AG, Nagraj HS et al. Effects of human growth hormone in men over 60 years old. *New England Journal of Medicine* 1990;323:1–6.

28. Vijayakumar A, Yakar S, LeRoith D. The intricate role of growth hormone in metabolism. *Frontiers in Endocrinology* 2011;2(32):1–21.

29. Clemmons DR. The relative roles of growth hormone and IGF-1 in controlling insulin sensitivity. *Journal of Clinical Investigation* 2004;113(1):25–27.

30. Olleros Santos-Ruiz M, Sadaba MC, Martin-Estal I et al. The single IGF-1 partial deficiency is responsible for mitochondrial dysfunction and is restored by IGF-1 replacement therapy. *Growth Hormone & IGF Research* 2017;35:21–32.

31. Moreau OK, Cortet-Rudelli C, Yollin E et al. Growth hormone replacement therapy in patients with traumatic brain injury. *Journal of Neurotrauma* 2013;30(11):998–1006.

32. Handler MZ, Ross AL, Shiman MI et al. Potential role of human growth hormone in melanoma growth promotion. *Archives of Dermatology* 2012;148(10):1179–82.

33. Ma J, Pollak MN, Giovannucci E et al. Prospective study of colorectal cancer risk in men and plasma levels of insulin-like growth factor (IGF)-1 and IGF-binding protein-3. *Journal of the National Cancer Institute* 1999;91(7):620–5.

34. Ameri P, Giusti A, Boschetti M et al. Interactions between vitamin D and IGF-1: from physiology to clinical practice. *Clinical Endocrinology* 2013;79(4):457–63.

35. Godfrey RJ, Madgwick Z, Whyte P. The exercise-induced growth hormone response in athletes. *Sports Medicine* 2003;33(8):599–613.

36. Liu H, Bravata DM, Olkin I et al. Systematic review: the effects of growth hormone on athletic performance. *Annals of Internal Medicine* 2008;148(10):747–58.

37. Meinhardt U, Nelson AE, Hansen JL et al. The effects of growth hormone on body composition and physical performance in recreational athletes: a randomized trial. *Annals of Internal Medicine* 2010;152(9):568–77.

38. Hintz RL. Growth hormone: uses and abuses. *BMJ* 2004;328(7445):907–8.

39. Bartke A. Growth hormone and aging: a challenging controversy. *Clinical Interventions in Aging* 2008;3(4):659–65.

40. Milman S, Huffman DM, Barzilai N. The somatotropic axis in human aging: framework for the current state of knowledge and future research. *Cell Metabolism* 2016;23(6):980–9.

41. Guadalupe-Grau A, Carniocero JA, Losa-Reyna J et al. Endocrinology of aging from a muscle point of view: results from the Toledo study for healthy aging. *Journal of the American Medical Directors Association* 2017;18(3):234–9.

42. Xu Y, Nadungadi TP, Zhu L et al. Distinct hypothalamic neurons mediate estrogenic effects on energy homeostasis and reproduction. *Cell Metabolism* 2011;14(4):453–65.

43. Peretz J, Pekosz A, Lane AP et al. Estrogenic compounds reduce influenza A virus replication in primary human nasal epithelial cells derived from female, but not male, donors. *American Journal of Physiology—Lung Cellular and Molecular Physiology* 2016;310(5):L415–25.

44. Albert K, Hiscox J, Boyd B et al. Estrogen enhances hippocampal gray-matter volume in young and older postmenopausal women: a prospective dose-response study. *Neurobiology of Aging* 2017;56:1–6.

45. Wu MV, Tollkuhn J. Estrogen receptor alpha is required in GABAergic, but not glutamatergic, neurons to masculinize behavior. *Hormones and Behavior* 2017;95:3–12.

46. Lei P, Xu Y, Gan Y et al. Estrogen enhances matrix synthesis in nucleus pulposus cell through the estrogen receptor beta-p38 MAPK pathway. *Cellular Physiology and Biochemistry* 2016;39:2216–26.

47. Lou C, Chen H, Mei L et al. Association between menopause and lumbar degenerative disc degeneration: an MRI study of 1,566 women and 1,382 men. *Menopause* 2017;doi:10.1097/GME.0000000000000902 (epub ahead of print).

48. Pinkerton JV, Abraham L, Bushmakin AG et al. Relationship between changes in vasomotor symptoms and changes in menopause-specific quality of life and sleep parameters. *Menopause* 2016;23(10):1060–6.

49. Writing Group for the Women's Health Initiative Investigators. Risks and benefits of estrogen plus progestin in healthy postmenopausal women: principal results from the Women's Health Initiative randomized controlled trial. *JAMA* 2002;288(3):321–33.

50. Sarrel PM, Njike VY, Vinante V et al. The mortality toll of estrogen avoidance: an analysis of excess deaths among hysterectomized women aged 50 to 59 years. *American Journal of Public Health* 2013;103(9):1583–8.

51. Zimmerman MA, Hutson DD, Trimmer EH et al. Long- but not short-term estradiol treatment induces renal damage in midlife ovariectomized Long-Evans rats. *American Journal of Physiology—Renal Physiology* 2017;312(2):F305–11.

52. Ez-Zoubir A, Pisani DF. Control of bone and fat mass by oxytocin. *Hormone Molecular Biology and Clinical Investigation* 2016:28(2):95–104.

53. Pedersen CA, Prange AJ. Induction of maternal behavior in virgin rats after intracerebroventricular administration of oxytocin. *Proceedings of the National Academy of Sciences* 1979;76(12):6661–5.

54. Zak PJ, Kurzban R, Matzner WT. Oxytocin is associated with human trustworthiness. *Hormones and Behavior* 2005;48(5):522–7.

55. Ebner NC, Horta M, Lin T et al. Oxytocin modulates meta-mood as a function of age and sex. *Frontiers in Aging Neuroscience* 2015;7:175–94.

56. Theofanopoulou C. Implications of oxytocin in human linguistic cognition: from genome to phenome. *Frontiers in Neuroscience* 2016;10:271.

57. Neumann ID, Slattery DA. Oxytocin in general anxiety and social fear: a translational approach. *Biological Psychiatry* 2016;79(3):213–21.

58. Marlin BJ, Mitre M, D'amour JA et al. Oxytocin enables maternal behavior by balancing cortical inhibition. *Nature* 2015;520(7548):499–504.

59. Owen SF, Tuncdemir SN, Bader PL et al. Oxytocin enhances hippocampal spike transmission by modulating fast-spiking interneurons. *Nature* 2013;500(7463):458–62.

60. Wang H, Duclot F, Liu Y et al. Histone deacetylase inhibitors facilitate partner preference formation in female prairie voles. *Nature Neuroscience* 2013;16(7):919–24.

61. Ez-Zoubir A. Control of bone and fat mass by oxytocin. 2016:95–104.

62. Houshmand F, Faghihi M, Zahediasl S. Role of atrial natriuretic peptide in oxytocin induced cardioprotection. *Heart, Lung & Circulation* 2015;24(1):86–93.

63. Elabd C, Cousin W, Upadhyayula P et al. Oxytocin is an age-specific circulating hormone that is necessary for muscle maintenance and regeneration. *Nature Communications* 2014;10(5):4082.

64. Ez-Zoubir A. Control of bone and fat mass by oxytocin. 2016:95–104.

65. Kassotis CD, Hoffman K, Stapleton HM. Characterization of adipogenic activity of house dust extracts and semi-volatile indoor contaminants in 3T3-L1 cells. *Environmental Science & Technology* 2017;51(15):8735–45.

66. McCullough ME, Churchland PS, Mendez AJ. Problems with measuring peripheral oxytocin: can the data on oxytocin and human behavior be trusted? *Neuroscience & Biobehavioral Reviews* 2013;37(8):1485–92.

67. Wu L, Meng J, Shen Q et al. Caffeine inhibits hypothalamic A1R to excite oxytocin neuron and ameliorate dietary obesity in mice. *Nature Communications* 2017;8:15904.

## CHAPTER 15

1. Justice J, Miller JD, Newman JC et al. Frameworks for proof-of-concept clinical trials of interventions that target fundamental aging processes. *Journals of Gerontology. Series A, Biological Sciences and Medical Sciences* 2016;71(11):1415–23.

2. Vaiserman AM, Luschak OV, Koliada AK. Anti-aging pharmacology: promises and pitfalls. *Ageing Research Reviews* 2016;31:9–35.

3. Toussant O, Dumont P, Remacle J et al. Stress-induced premature senescence or stress-induced senescence-like phenotype: one in vivo reality, two possible definitions? *Scientific World Journal* 2002;2:230–47.

4. Baker DJ, Wijshake T, Tchkonia T et al. Clearance of p16$^{Ink-4a}$-positive senescent cells delays ageing-associated disorders. *Nature* 2011;479:232–6.

5. Baker DJ, Childs BG, Durik M et al. Naturally occurring p16$^{Ink4a}$-positive cells shorten healthy lifespan. *Nature* 2016;530:184–9.

6. Stewart-Ornstein J, Lahav G. P53 dynamics in response to DNA damage vary across cell lines and are shaped by efficiency of DNA repair and activity of the kinase ATM. *Science Signaling* 2017;10(476):eaah6671.

7. Demir O, Ieong PU, Amaro RE. Full-length p53 tetramer bound to DNA and its quaternary dynamics. *Oncogene* 2017;36(10):1451–60.

8. Baar MP, Brandt RMC, Putavet DA et al. Targeted apoptosis of senescent cells restores tissue homeostasis in response to chemotoxicity and aging. *Cell* 2017;169(1):132–47.

9. Childs BG, Baker DJ, Wijshake T et al. Senescent intimal foam cells are deleterious at all stages of atherosclerosis. *Science* 2016;354(6311):472–7.

10. Jeon OH, Kim C, Laberge RM et al. Local clearance of senescent cells attenuates the development of post-traumatic osteoarthritis and creates a pro-regenerative environment. *Nature Medicine* 2017: doi:10.1038/nm.4324

11. Jin J, Tao J, Gu X et al. P16$^{Ink4a}$ deletion ameliorated renal tubulointerstitial injury in a stress-induced premature senescence model of Bmi-1 deficiency. *Scientific Reports* 2017;7:7502.

12. Xu M, Palmer AK, Ding H et al. Targeting senescent cells enhances adipogenesis and metabolic function in old age. *eLife* 2015;2:e129997.

13. Kirkland JL, Tchkonia T. Clinical strategies and animal models for developing senolytic agents. *Experimental Gerontology* 2015;68:19–25.

14. Kirkland JL, Tchkonia T: Cellular senescence: a translational perspective. *EBio-Medicine* 2017;21:21–28.

15. Coyle C, Cafferty FH, Vale C et al. Metformin as an adjuvant treatment for cancer: a systematic review and meta-analysis. *Annals of Oncology* 2016;27(12):2184–95.

16. Barzalai N, Crandall JP, Kritchevsky SB et al. Metformin as a tool to target aging. *Cell Metabolism* 2016;23(6):1060–5.

17. Liu B, Fan Z, Edgerton SM et al. Potent anti-proliferative effects of metformin on trastuzumab-resistant breast cancer cells via inhibition of erbB2/IGF-1 receptor interactions. *Cell Cycle* 2011;10(17):2959–66.

18. Nair V, Sreevalsan S, Basha R et al. Mechanism of metformin-dependent inhibition of mammalian target of rapamycin (mTOR) and Ras activity in pancreatic cancer: role of specificity protein (Sp) transcription factors. *Journal of Biological Chemistry* 2014;289(40):27692–701.

19. Bridges HR, Jones AJ, Pollak MN et al. Effects of metformin and other biguanides on oxidative phosphorylation in mitochondria. *Biochemical Journal* 2014;462(Pt. 3):475–87.

20. Duca FA, Cote CD, Rasmussen BA et al. Metformin activates a duodenal AMPK-dependent pathway to lower hepatic glucose production in rats. *Nature Medicine* 2015;21(5):506–11.

21. Algire C, Moiseeva O, Deschenes-Simard X et al. Metformin reduces endogenous reactive oxygen species and associated DNA damage. *Cancer Prevention Research* 2012;5(4):536–43.

## CHAPTER 16

1. Boutilier JA. METEI: a Canadian medical expedition to Easter Island, 1964-1965 [part I]. *Rapa Nui Journal* 1992;6(2):21–33.

2. Boutilier JA. METEI: a Canadian medical expedition to Easter Island, 1964-1965 [part II]. *Rapa Nui Journal* 1992;6(3):45–53.

3. Vezina C, Kudelski A, Sehgal SN. Rapamycin (AY-22,989), a new antifungal antibiotic. I. taxonomy of the producing streptomycete and isolation of the active principle. *Journal of Antibiotics* 1975;28(10):721–6.

4. Sehgal SN. Sirolimus: its discovery, biological properties, and mechanism of action. *Transplantation Proceedings* 2003;35(3 Suppl.):7S–14S.
5. https://www.justice.gov/opa/pr/wyeth-pharmaceuticals-agrees-pay-4909-million -marketing-prescription-drug-rapamune-unapproved
6. https://www.justice.gov/usao-ma/pr/wyeth-and-pfizer-agree-pay-7846-million -resolve-lawsuit-alleging-wyeth-underpaid-drug
7. Heitman J, Movva R, Hall MN. Targets for cell cycle arrest by the immunosuppressant rapamycin in yeast. *Science* 1991;253(5022):905–9.
8. De Magalhaes JP, Wuttke D, Wood SH et al. Genome-environment interactions that modulate aging: powerful targets for drug recovery. *Pharmacological Reviews* 2012;64(1):88–101.
9. Kim YC, Guan KL. mTOR: a pharmacologic target for autophagy regulation. *Journal of Clinical Investigation* 2015; 125(1):25–32.
10. Laberge RM, Sun Y, Orjalo AV et al. mTOR regulates the pro-tumorigenic senescence-associated secretory phenotype by promoting IL1A translation. *Nature Cell Biology* 2015;17(8):1049–61.
11. Walker NM, Belloi EA, Stuckey L et al. Mechanistic target of rapamycin complex 1 (mTORC1) and mTORC2 as key signaling intermediates in mesenchymal cell activation. *Journal of Biological Chemistry* 2016;291(12):6262–71.
12. Harrison DE, Strong R, Sharp ZD et al. Rapamycin fed late in life extends lifespan in genetically heterogeneous mice. *Nature* 2009;460:392–5.
13. Herranz N, Gallage S, Mellone M et al. mTOR regulates MAPKAPK2 translation to control senescence-associated secretory phenotype. *Nature Cell Biology* 2015;17(9):1205–17.
14. Correia-Melo C, Marques FDM, Nelson JF et al. Mitochondria are required for pro-ageing features of the senescent phenotype. *EMBO Journal* 2016;35(7):724–42.
15. Betz C, Hall MN. Where is mTOR and what is it doing there? *Journal of Cell Biology* 2013;203(4):563–74.
16. Johnson SC, Kaeberlein M. Rapamycin in aging and disease: maximizing efficacy while minimizing side effects. *Oncotarget* 216;7(29):44876–8.
17. Harrison DE, Strong R, Sharp ZD et al. Rapamycin fed late in life extends lifespan in genetically heterogenous mice. *Nature* 2009;460(7253):392–5.
18. Siddiqui A, Bhaumik D, Chinta SJ et al. Mitochondrial quality control via the PGC1-TFEB signaling pathway is compromised by parkin Q311X mutation but independently restored by rapamycin. *Journal of Neuroscience* 2015;35(37):12833.

19. Luo D, Ren H, Li T et al. Rapamycin reduces severity of senile osteoporosis by activating osteocyte autophagy. *Osteoporosis International* 2016;27(3):1093–101.

20. Seto B. Rapamycin and mTOR: a serendipitous discovery and implications for breast cancer. *Clinical and Translational Medicine* 2012;1(1):29.

21. Choi J, Kim H, Bae YK et al. REP1 modulates autophagy and macropinocytosis to enhance cancer cell survival. *International Journal of Molecular Sciences* 2017;18(9):pii:E1866.

22. Ross C, Salmon A, Strong R et al. Metabolic consequences of long-term rapamycin exposure on common marmoset monkeys (*Callithrix jacchus*). *Aging* 2015;7(11):964–73.

23. Mannick JB, Del Giudice G, Lattanzi M et al. mTOR inhibition improves immune function in the elderly. *Science Translational Medicine* 2014;6(268):268ra179.

24. Riera CE, Dillin A. Emerging role of sensory perception in aging and metabolism. *Trends in Endocrinology and Metabolism* 2016;27(5):294–303.

25. Riera CE, Huising MO, Follett P et al. TRPV1 pain receptors regulate longevity and metabolism by neuropeptide signaling. *Cell* 2014;157(5):1023–36.

26. Steculorum SM, Bruning J. Die another day: a painless path to longevity. *Cell* 2014;157(5):1004–6.

27. Sonowal R, Swimm A, Sahoo A et al. Indoles from commensal bacteria extend healthspan. *PNAS* 2017;114(36):E7506–15; http://www.pnas.org/content/early/2017/08/15/1706464114.abstract.

## CHAPTER 17

1. Munro D, Treberg JR. A radical shift in perspective: mitochondria as regulators of reactive oxygen species. *Journal of Experimental Biology* 2017;220(7):1170–80.

2. Bulka CM, Davis MA, Karagas MR et al. The unintended consequences of a gluten-free diet. *Epidemiology* 2017;28(3):e24–5.

3. Dellinger RW, Garcia AMG, Meyskens FL. Differences in the glucuronidation of resveratrol and pterostilbene: altered enzyme specificity and potential gender differences. *Drug Metabolism and Pharmacokinetics* 2014;29(2):112–9.

4. Li J, Bonkowski MS, Moniot S et al. A conserved NAD+ binding pocket that regulates protein-protein interactions during aging. *Science* 2017;355(6331):1312–7.

5. Moore AC, Patel AV, Matthews CE. Leisure time physical activity of moderate to vigorous intensity and mortality: a large pooled cohort analysis. *PLOS Medicine* 2012;9(11):e1001335.

6. Travison TG, Araujo AB, O'Donnell AB et al. A population-level decline in serum testosterone levels in American men. *Journal of Clinical Endocrinology and Metabolism* 2007;92(1):196–202.

7. Bhasin S. Secular decline in male reproductive function: is manliness threatened? *Journal of Clinical Endocrinology and Metabolism* 2007;92(1):44–5.

8. Elabd C, Cousin W, Upadhyayula P et al. Oxytocin is an age-specific circulating hormone that is necessary for muscle maintenance and regeneration. *Nature Communications* 2014;5:4082.

# INDEX

Underscored page references indicate boxed text. **Boldface** references indicate illustrations.

## A

Adenosine triphosphate (ATP)
  body fat and, 72
  daily need for, 44
  energy from, 28, 51
  exercise and, 136
  iron and, 107
  mitochondrial dysfunction and, 35–36
  mTOR levels and, 99, 196–97
  muscular contractions and, **134**
  niacin and, 45
  production of, 28–31, **29–30**, 42–43
  riboflavin and, 117
Age-related macular degeneration (AMD),
  61–62
Aging. *See also* Longevity
  accelerating
    inflammation, 33, 36
    methylation, 14, 22, 26, 80
    obesity, 80
    protein consumption, 95, 99
  brain's resistance to, 22, 65
  mitochondria and, 43–44, 203–5
  scientific advancements in, 183–88,
    198–200, 203–5
  seven pathways of, 31–37, **38,** 204
    cellular senescence, 36–37
    deregulated nutrient sensing, 35
    DNA damage, 32
    epigenetic alterations, 33–34
    mitochondrial dysfunction, 35–36
    proteostasis, loss of, 34
    telomere erosion, 32–33
  slowing
    anti-aging drugs, 184–87, 187, 209–11
    (*see also* Rapamycin)
    exercise, 132, 132, 198
    hormones, 173–77
    social connections, 158–60, 166
    telomere length and, 32–33, 184
Alcohol, 108, 115–16, 170, 207
Alzheimer's disease, 34, 42, 81, 184
AMD, 61–62
Amino acids, 92–94
AMP-kinase (AMPK), 51, 136, 187
Anemia, 107, 120–21, 125
Antidepressants, 179, 210
Anti-inflammatories, 9, 108, 112
Antioxidants, 9, 42–43, 51–52, 112, 117,
  120, 184
Arthritis, 64, 186
Artificial sweeteners, 81–84
Ascorbic acid, 120–21
Aspartame, 82–83
Atherosclerosis, 76
Atkins Diet, 93
ATP. *See* Adenosine triphosphate
Autoimmune diseases, 7–8, 87
Autophagy
  brain health and, 34, 136
  improving with
    calorie-restriction (CR), 51
    exercise, 132
    rapamycin, 184, 195–97, **196**
  process of, 34, 184

# B

Bacteria, 24, 26, 39–40, 58–59, 199. *See also* Microbiome
B-cell activating factor (BAFF), 7–8
BDNF, 137, 143, 149
Biotin, 119
Blindness, 61–62, 116
Blood pressure, 85, 113
Blood sugar, 77, 83, 144
Blue zones, 3–18
  Ikaria, Greece, 10–12
  life span in, 4, 9, 18
  Loma Linda, California, 15–16
  Nicoya, Costa Rica, 12–15
  Okinawa, Japan, 8–10
  overview, 3–4, 8, 12, 18
  Sardinia, 4–8
Body fat, 50, 52–53, 72, 180, 180. *See also* Weight loss
Bone health
  exercise and, 144
  fractures, 144–45, 207
  oxytocin and, 180
  pH balance and, 94
  spine and, 177
  vegan diet and, 105
  vitamins and minerals for, 120–25
Boniva, 144
Bowman-Birk factors, 97–98, 107
Brain, 158–66. *See also* Dementia
  aging and, 22, 36, 65
  anatomy of, **159**
  energy requirements of, 50, 71, 151, **159**
  health of, 136–38, 160–65
  hormones and, 171–73, **172**
  injuries to, 175
  lactic acid and, 137, 161
  mitochondria in, 41, 43
  obesity and, 81
  stress and, 149–50
Brain-derived neurotrophic factor (BDNF), 137, 143, 149

# C

Caffeine, 33, 112–13, 198
Calcium, 94, 105, 125–26, 144–45, 207
Calorie restriction (CR), 49–56
  effects on
    dementia, 34
    diabetes, 51–52, 104
    inflammation, 52
    liver, 52–53
    metabolism, 45, 49–52, 50, 70–71
    NAD+ levels, 45, 47, 51–53

nutrient sensing, 35
  overweight, 53–55, 71, 209
  telomere length, 33
  4-hour rule and, 54–55, **55**
  history of, 49–50
  types of, 53–55, 56
Calorie-restriction mimetics, 53–54, 184–87, 187
Cancer
  causes of
    bacteria, 26
    diet, 82, 86, 96–97, 106–7, 127
    inheritance, 65
    senescent cells, 36, 185–86
    sunlight, 123–24
    telomere length, 21, 33
  DNA damage and, 48
  hormones and, 170, 175–79, 210
  prevention of, 142–43, 142, 187
  treatments for, 108, 153
  tumor-monitoring proteins, 32
Carbohydrates, 76, 86–90, 92. *See also specific foods*
Cardio (endurance) exercise, 6, 140–41, 208–9
Cardiovascular disease
  causes of, 177–78, 185, 206
  diet and, 73–77, 73
  fish oil supplementation and, 126
  genetic editing and, 65
  prevention of, 16, 105, 112, 144, 146
  salt and, 85
Cas enzymes, 58–62
Celiac disease, 87
Cellular respiration, 28–31, **29–30**
Cellular senescence, 36–37, 43–44, 73, 76–77, 145, 184–86, 206
Centenarians, 3, 8–9, 18
Cholesterol, 73–76, 73, 172, 206–7
Chromosomes, **25**, 25–27, 33, 155, 180. *See also* Telomere length
Chronic granulomatous disease, 63
Circadian rhythms, 45, 47, 54, **55**, 184
Cobalamin, 105, 119–20
Coffee, 112–13, 113, 128, 198, 207
Complex regional pain syndrome (CRPS), 121
Concentration, 163–64
Congenital cardiomyopathy, 64–65
Conserved transcriptional response to adversity (CTRA), 149–51
Cortisol, 52, 77
Cpf1, 62
CR. *See* Calorie restriction
Creativity and flow, 162–65
CRISPR gene editing. *See* Genetic editing

CrossFit, 145–46, 208
CRPS, 121
CTRA, 149–51
Cyclamates, 82

# D

Dairy products, 59, 105
Death. *See* Mortality risk
Dementia
  causes of, 34, 42, 81, 83
  prevention of, 9, 34, 113–14, 161–62
Depression, 150, 153
DHA, 126–27
Diabetes
  causes of, 35, 79–80, 96–97, 206
  prevention of, 9, 104, 112, 144
  treatment of, 51–52, 187
Diet, 69–91. *See also* Calorie restriction (CR);
    Weight loss
  adaptability to changes in, 71–72
  artificial sweeteners, 81–84
  fat in (*see* Dietary fat)
  guidelines and recommendations for,
    89–90, 92, 205–8
  heart disease and, 73, 73–77
  high-protein (*see* Protein)
  low-fat, 74, 89, 116, 173
  overview, 91
  salt and, 84–86
  sugar and, 77–81, 78
  wheat and, 86–89
Dietary fat
  guidelines and requirements for, 72, 90, 92
  hormones and, 77
  low-fat diet and, 74, 89, 116, 173
  obesity and, 80
  saturated fat, 73, 73–76, 90, 206
  studies on, 73–77, 89
  testosterone and, 77, 172–73
  types of, 73
Diet-induced thermogenesis (DIT), 93
Disease resistance, 7–8
DNA. *See also* Genetic editing; Methylation
  chromosomes and, 25–26, 25
  damage to, 24, 32, 48
  environmental effects on, 20–22, 26, 204
  errors in replication, 27
  exercise and, 133–34, 145
  human genome, 24, 25
  mitochondrial DNA (mtDNA), 36, 40–43,
    46, 136, 184
  repairing, 47, 118, 208
  senescence and, 185
  stress and, 32, 150

tai chi and, 155
ultraviolet radiation and, 123
volume of, 27

# E

Effexor, 179
Emotional connections, 158–60, 166
Energy
  aging and, 203–4
  carbohydrates for, 99
  metabolism and, 27–31, 29–30
  mitochondria and, 40–42
  niacin for, 118
Epigenetics, 12, 21–22, 33–34, 145, 204
Equal, 82–83
ERRalpha (estrogen-related receptor alpha),
    137
Escitalopram, 179
Essential fatty acids, 72–73, 77, 105–6, 126–27
Estrogen, 169–70, 177–79, 209–10
Estrogen-related receptor alpha (ERRalpha),
    137
Exercise, 131–47. *See also specific types*
  benefits of
    brain health, 136–38
    cholesterol levels, 76
    depression reduction, 150
    hormones, 77, 173
    longevity, 131–32, 132, 142, 198
    metabolism, 133
    telomere length, 33, 135
    vitamin D levels, 124, 143
  calorie restriction (CR) and, 71
  medication vs., 137
  muscular contractions and, 133–35, **134**
  NAD+ levels and, 45, 47, 136
  overview, 131–32, 139, 140–41, 148
  recommendations for, 208–9
  weight loss and, 70–72, 144, 209
Experiential technology (XTech), 162

# F

FAD, 117
Fasting, 49–50, 50, 52–55, 56, 136–37. *See also*
    Calorie restriction (CR)
Fasting-mimetic diet, 53–54
Fatigue, 107, 153, 164–65
FDA
  on anti-aging medications, 187
  on artificial sweeteners, 82, 84
  dietary recommendations of, 74
  on gene editing, 59
  on rapamycin, 194

FDA (cont.)
  safrole, ban on, 108
  supplement monitoring and, 127
  on trans fats, 76
Feast-or-famine fasting, 53
Fertility, 16, 106
Fiber, 104
Fibromyalgia, 154
Fish oil, 126–27
Flavin adenine dinucleotide (FAD), 117
Flavonoids, 198, 207
FNDC5, 137, 143
Fountain plan, 203–12
  diet recommendations, 205–8
  drug information, 209–11
  exercise recommendations, 208–9
  overview, 212
  science and, 203–5
4-hour rule, 54–55, **55**. See also Calorie
  restriction (CR)

**G**

Gender. See also Hormones
  essential fatty acid needs and, 72, 77
  iron stores and, 124–25
  longevity and, 5, 13, 15
  vegetarian diets and, 102
Gene expression, 22, 80, 134, 152
Genes. See also Methylation; Telomere length
  adaptability of, 72, 80
  aging and, 12, 21, 204
  for disease resistance, 7–8
  environment and, 19–22, **20**, 33
  exercise and, 133–34, 143, 145
  high cholesterol and, 206–7
  human genome, 24, 25
  inflammation and, 33
  inherited traits, 33, 41, 65
  mind-body interventions and, 151–52, 152
  vegetarian diets and, 106–7
  vitamin D deficiency and, 124
Gene splicing, 59–61, **60**
Genetic editing, 57–66
  age-related macular degeneration (AMD)
    and, 61–62
  aging and, 63–65
  CRISPR origins, 58
  ethics of, 63–65
  gene splicing and, 59–61, **60**
  history of, 58–59
  regulation of, 65
  stem cell research and, 62–63
  timeline of research, 66

GH. See Growth hormone
Glucophage, 186–87, 187
Glucose, 28, **29**, 77, 79, 175
Gluten, 86–89, 87, 207
Growth hormone (GH), 169–70, 174–76, 210
Gut flora. See Microbiome

**H**

Happiness, 158–61
Heart health. See also Cardiovascular disease
  cardiomyopathy and, 64–65
  heart attack causes, 43, 85
  high-protein diets and, 95
  Mediterranean diet for, 76–77
  mitochondria and, 41, 43
  running and, 141–42
High-intensity interval training (HIIT), 145–47
High-intensity resistance training, 77
High-protein diets, 71–72, 93–95, 96, 100,
  206. See also Protein
Hormones, 169–82. See also specific hormones
  aging and, 173–77
  cancer and, 170, 175–78, 210
  dietary fat and, 77
  for hunger signals, 53
  overview, 169–70, 182
  recommendations for, 209–11
Human genome, 24, 25
Human growth hormone (GH). See Growth
  hormone
Hunger signals, 53, 85, 93
Hunter-gatherer tribes, 70, 77–78
Hypertension, 85

**I**

IGF-1. See Insulin-like growth factor-1
IL-6, 142, 153
IL-32, 80
Immune system, 7–8, 24, 58, 142, 197–98
Inflammation
  causes of
    celiac disease, 87
    cellular remnants, 36
    diet, 86, 97–98, 104, 106–7
    senescent cells, 185, 206
    stress, 150
    tumor-monitoring proteins, lack of, 32
  decreasing with
    calorie restriction (CR), 52, 55
    coffee, 112–13
    curcumin, 9
    exercise, 143

polyphenols, 108
yoga, 153
effects of, 31, 33, 36, 73, 76
obesity and, 80
SIRT6 and regulation of, 46
Inherited traits, 33, 41, 65
Insulin-like growth factor-1 (IGF-1)
Alzheimer's disease and, 34
calorie restriction (CR) and, 54
exercise and, 142, 143
high-protein diets and, 95–99, 206
hormones and, 175–76
Metformin for, 187
Parkinson's disease and, 42
Insulin resistance, 76, 79–80, 112, 136
Interleukin-6 (IL-6), 142, 153
Interleukin-32 (IL-32), 80
Intermittent fasting, 53
Iodine, 86
Iron, 107, 124–25, 125

**K**

Kidney health, 23, 94, 179, 184, 206
Krebs cycle, 29–31, **29**, 35, 51

**L**

Lactic acid, 31, 117, 133, 137, 161
Lectins, 109
Leptin, 53, 72
Lexapro, 179
Life in the Box, 208
Liver
diet and, 52–53, 80, 112, 115
function of, 23, 52, 116, 122
hormones and, 171, 173–75
IGF-1 levels and, 54
SIRT3 levels and, 46
Longevity. See also Aging; Mortality risk
in blue zones, 4, 9, 18
centenarians and, 3, 8–9, 18
gender and, 5, 13, 15
geographical zones of (blue zones), 3–4
height and, 5
increasing with
calorie-restricted diets, 45, 55
coffee, 112
exercise for, 131–32, 132, 147, 198
meaning in life, 160–61
running, 142
tai chi, 154
vegetarian/vegan diets and, 102, 104
Low-fat diets, 74, 89, 116, 173

**M**

Meaning in life, 160–61
Meat. See Protein
Mechanistic target of rapamycin (mTOR)
natural regulators of, 198, 204
protein consumption and, 98–99
suppressing, 35, 187, 187, 195–98, **196**
Meditation, 151–52, 152, 164
Mediterranean diet, 76–77
Melatonin, 184
Men. See Gender; Testosterone
Menopause, 177–79
Metabolism
adaptability of, 70–71, 94
aging and, 37, 38, 203–4
circadian rhythms and, 54
energy for, 28, 93
improving with
calorie restriction (CR), 45, 49–52, 50, 70–71
exercise, 133
pterostilbene, 115
proteostasis, loss of, 34
Metformin, 186–87, 187
Methylation
aging and stress caused by, 14, 21, 26, 80
defined, 14
improving, 114, 133–35, 145, 153, 155
as measure of biological age, 13, 21–22, 31, 33
obesity and, 80
Microbiome
adaptability of, 72
effect of
artificial sweeteners, 83
celiac disease, 87
protein consumption, 97
vegetarian diet, 104
function of, 24
importance of, 205
Micronutrients, 115–26
MiDAS, 43–44
Mind-body interventions, 150–52, 152
Mind games and exercises, 161–62
Mitochondria, 39–48
aging and, 43–44, 203–5
antioxidants of, 42–43
calorie restriction (CR) and, 50–51
damage to, 14
dysfunction, aging and, 35–36
exercise and, 147
fission and fusion of, 41–43, 136
function of, 28–30, **29–30**

Mitochondria (*cont.*)
nicotinamide adenine dinucleotide
(NAD+) and, 44–47
properties of, 39–41, <u>48</u>
Mitochondrial DNA (mtDNA), 36, 40–43,
46, 136, 184
Mitochondrial dysfunction-associated
senescence (MiDAS), 43–44
Mitochondrial reactive oxidative species
(mtROS), 50
Mortality risk
carbohydrates and, 89–90
cholesterol levels and, 75
coffee and, 112
dietary fats and, 75–76, 89
exercise and, 142, 147
high-protein diets and, 95–97
obesity and, 80
salt and, 85
mtDNA. *See* Mitochondrial DNA
mTOR. *See* Mechanistic target of rapamycin
Multiple sclerosis, 138
Muscles
brain and, 138, <u>161</u>, 163
effect of
diet, 77, 99, 105
exercise, 71, 133–35, **134**, 142, 209
methylation, 14, 80
vitamins and minerals, 122–25
growth hormone (GH) and, 175–76
oxytocin and, 180
soreness of, 31
strength training for, 140–41, 143–45
Muscular dystrophy, 62

**N**
NAAD, 118
NAD+. *See* Nicotinamide adenine
dinucleotide
NADH, 44, 47
NADP, 117
NAMPT, 44–45, 51
NASA Twins Study, 19–22, **20**, 24
NgAgo, 62
Niacin, 45, 47, 117–18
Nicotinamide adenine dinucleotide (NAD+)
aging and, 35–36, 52, 207–8
calorie restriction (CR) and, 45, 47, 51–53
DNA repair and, 32, <u>47</u>
exercise and, 45, 47, 136
Krebs cycle and, 28–30, **31**
MiDAS cells and, 44
mitochondria and, 44–47, 205

niacin and, 117–18
riboflavin and, 117
Nicotinamide adenine dinucleotide
hydrogen (NADH), 44, 47
Nicotinamide adenine dinucleotide
phosphate (NADP), 117
Nicotinamide mononucleotide (NMN), 45,
47, 118
Nicotinamide riboside (NR), 47, 118, 208
Nicotinamide salvage pathway, 44–47
Nicotinic acid adenine dinucleotide
(NAAD), 118
Nitrates/nitrites, 95
NMN, 45, 47, 118
NR, 47, 118, 208
Nuclear respiratory factor 1 (NRF-1), 135–36
NutraSweet, 82–83
Nutrient sensing, 35

**O**
Obesity
causes of
deregulated nutrient sensing, 35
diet, 69, 76, 79–80, 88, 206
sedentary lifestyle, 70
effect on
hormones, 170, 173
hypertension, 85
insulin resistance, 80
Oxidative stress, 52, 114, 155, 184
Oxytocin, 169–70, 179–81, 210–11

**P**
Pain, 153–54, 190, 198
Paleolithic Diet, 71–72, 93, <u>96</u>
Pancreas, 43, 80
Pantothenic acid, 118–19
Parathyroid hormones, 105, **122**, 125, 144
Parkinson's disease, 42, 113, 184
Paroxetine, 179
PARPs. *See* Poly ADP-ribose polymerases
Partially hydrogenated oils, 73
Paxil, 179
PGC-1 alpha, 136–37, 142–44
pH levels, 94, 99
Phytates, 107–8
Phytochemicals, 108–9, 112, 116
Pilates, 155–56
Pituitary gland, **172**
Plant-based diets, 34, 95–96, 206. *See also*
Vegetarian/vegan diets
Pluripotent stem cells, 63–64

P90X exercise program, 146
Poly ADP-ribose polymerases (PARPs),
    44–46, 47, 51, 118, 205, 208
Polyphenols, 108, 112, 114, 198
Polyunsaturated fat, 74–75
Pregnant women, 105, 116
Productivity, 163–65
Prolia, 144
Protein, 92–100
    dietary guidelines for, 92
    effect on body, 94–95, 99
    high-protein diets, 71–72, 93–95, 96, 100, 206
    IGF-1 levels and, 96–99
    metabolizing, 93–94
    studies on, 95–98
Proteostasis, loss of, 34
Pterostilbene, 115, 207
PureVia, 84
Purpose in life, sense of, 158–61
Pyridoxine, 119
Pyruvate, 44

Q
Qigong, 154–55

R
Rapamune, 194–95
Rapamycin
    benefits and effects of, 35, 184, 197
    development of, 193–95
    discovery of, 189–93
    mTOR and, 195–97, 196
Reactive oxygen species (ROS), 42–43, 51–52,
    136
Recovery, 164–65
Relaxation response, 151
Resveratrol, 108, 115, 207
Retinol, 116
Riboflavin, 117
RNA, 27, 40–41, 52, 62–63, 77, 109
Rockefeller Foundation Sardinian Project, 7
Running, 141–42

S
Saccharin, 81–82
Salt, 84–86, 206
Saturated fat, 73, 73–76, 90, 206
Scientific advancements in aging studies,
    183–88, 198–200, 203–5. See also
    Rapamycin
Sedentary lifestyle, 70, 135, 169

Seizures, 49–50
Senolytic medications, 36, 76, 184–86
Sensory receptors, 198–99
Seventh-Day Adventist (SDA), 15–16, 103–5
Sex, 173–74, 209
Sirtuin (SIRT) protein deacetylases
    caloric restriction and, 51–52
    function of, 45
    improving, 108, 114, 136
    melatonin and, 184
    metformin and, 187
Skin health, 116, 123–24
Smoking, 26, 79, 116, 170
Social connections, 158–60, 166
Spine health, 177
Splenda, 83
Statins, 76, 207
Stem cells, 32–33, 36, 62–65, 64, 116
Stevia, 83–84
Strength training, 140–41, 143–45
Stress, 149–57
    DNA damage and, 32, 150
    genes and, 26
    methylation and, 14, 21, 26, 80
    mitochondria, response to, 43
    reducing with
        meditation, 151–52, 152
        oxytocin, 180
        Pilates, 155–56
        tai chi, 154–55
        yoga, 152–54
    telomere length and, 21
Stroke, 74, 83, 85
Sucralose, 83
Sugar, 77–81, 79, 206. See also Glucose
Supplements, 111–28. See also Hormones
    coffee, 112–13, 128, 207
    fish oil and fatty acids, 126–27
    micronutrients, 115–26 (see also specific
        vitamins and minerals)
    for NAD+, 47
    resveratrol and pterostilbene, 115
    tea, 113–14, 113, 198, 207
Sweet-N-Low, 82

T
Tai chi, 150, 154–55, 209
TALENs, 61
Tea, 113–14, 113, 198, 207
Telomerase, 21, 32–33, 151, 184
Telomere length
    cell death and, 21
    defined, 13–14

Telomere length (*cont.*)
  environmental effects on, 21, 204
  erosion, aging and, 32–33, 184
  exercise and, 33, 135
  as measure of biological age, 13, 31
  mind-body interventions and, 151
  SIRT6 and regulation of, 46
Testosterone
  aging and, 169–70
  effects of
    cholesterol, 73, 206
    dietary fat, 77, 172–73
    exercise, 143
    stress, 21
    supplementation, 171, 173
  production of, 171–73, **172**
  recommendations for, 173, 210
Thiamin, 116–17
Thyroid, 86. *See also* Parathyroid hormones
Time-restricted feeding
  benefits of
    dementia prevention, 34
    nutrient sensing, 35
    weight loss, 54, 209
  4-hour rule for, 54–55, **55**
  overview, 56
Trace metals, 125–26
Transcription activator-like effector
    nucleases (TALENs), 61
Trans fats, 73–74, 76
TRPV-1, 198–99
Truvia, 84
Tryptophan, 45
T25 exercise program, 208
Turmeric, 9, 108

**U**

Unfolded protein response, 40, 47
Unsaturated fat, 53, 73–74, 90
Urea, 85
Uridine, 52–53
Urine, 94

**V**

Vascular endothelial growth factor (VEGF),
    61–62
Vascular system, 43
Vegetarian/vegan diets, 101–10
  effects on
    cardiovascular health, 16, 105
    diabetes, 104
    genetics, 106–7

  longevity, 102, 104
  weight, 15–16
  history of, 102
  nutritional needs and, 105–7, 116, 120, 206
  overview, 110
  variations in, 101, 105
VEGF, 61–62
Venlafaxine, 179
Vitamin A, 115
Vitamin B$_1$, 116–17
Vitamin B$_2$, 117
Vitamin B$_3$, 45, 47, 117–18
Vitamin B$_5$, 118–19
Vitamin B$_6$, 119
Vitamin B$_7$, 119
Vitamin B$_{12}$, 105, 119–20
Vitamin C, 120–21, 207
Vitamin D
  body's production of, 121–24, **122**
  for bone fractures, 145
  deficiencies in, 206
  exercise and, 124, 143
  IGF-1 and, 176
  supplements of, 124
  vegetarian diets and, 105

**W**

Weight loss. *See also* Body fat
  artificial sweeteners and, 83
  calorie restriction (CR) and, 53–55, 71,
    209
  exercise and, 70–72, 144, 209
  high-protein diets and, 93–95
  vegetarian diet and, 15–16
Weight resistance exercises, 140–41, 143–45
Wheat, 86–89, 87, 207
Whole30 Diet, 93
Wine, 108, 115
Women. *See* Estrogen; Gender

**X**

XTech (experiential technology), 162

**Y**

Yamanaka factors, 64
Yoga, 132, 141, 150–54, 209

**Z**

Zinc, 105, 116, 125–26
Zinc finger nuclease (ZFN), 61